Notes in Urgent Care

A Course Companion and Practical Guide

Notes in Urgent Care

A Course Companion and Practical Guide

MARTIN McGRATH FRCGP FFMLM MBChB MRAeS DCH DAvMED DipUMC DipIMC RCSEd MA

Honorary Professor, Faculty of Clinical and Biomedical Sciences
University of Central Lancashire, England
United Kingdom

Created to Support
University of Central Lancashire
Postgraduate Programmes

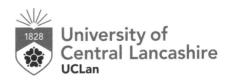

ISBN: 978-0-323-88407-5

Content Strategist: Alexandra Mortimer
Content Project Manager: Taranpreet Kaur
Design: Brian Salisbury
Marketing Manager: Deborah Watkins

Printed in India
Last digit is the print number: 9 8 7 6 5 4 3 2 1

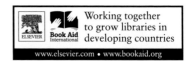

Working together
to grow libraries in
developing countries

www.elsevier.com • www.bookaid.org

CONTENTS

The provision of safe and effective urgent medical care has a positive effect on patient outcomes and has never been more important. Having (and being able to demonstrate) the correct knowledge, skills, competencies and attitudes to deliver this care should make a practitioner confident to do so in any setting, whether in remote or rural environments isolated from other expert help, or in urban environments where urgent medical care has become the 'front door' service for unscheduled care.

The University of Central Lancashire (UCLan) has established the National Centre for Remote and Rural Medicine, dedicated to providing the research and training required to equip health care practitioners to provide urgent medical care in any setting from remote mountains and deserts to oil platforms in the middle of raging seas and safe, warm consulting rooms within a city – indeed anywhere in the world.

This book serves as a framework to direct and support learning, both for students progressing through urgent medical care courses such as those run at UCLan or for those preparing for formal assessments in the area of urgent medical care such as the examinations run by the Royal College of Surgeons of Edinburgh; it is based on evidence that allows clinicians to work safely and is an invaluable resource.

Professor Cathy Jackson
Executive Dean, Faculty of Clinical and
Biomedical Sciences
University of Central Lancashire

The coupling of advances in medical technology and capability together with the introduction of 'time to treatment' targets has led to increasing secondary care demands. The resulting challenge is mirrored in primary care where the huge benefit derived from the aggressive management of long-term health conditions has reduced acute exacerbations and improved quality of life indicators but also led to reduced capacity to meet acute illness or 'same day' presentations. Urgent medical care (otherwise known as urgent and unscheduled care) offers a bridge between these spaces.

The delivery of effective urgent medical care comes from a blended, multidisciplinary response that can employ the latest technologies to identify serious conditions (such as ACS, sepsis, CVA and complicated injury) then start appropriate and timely treatment. Patients who access urgent medical care should have the confidence that there is no 'wrong' entry point to the system; trained clinicians will provide value-added steps wherever they attend, either resolving the complaint (and decompressing wider system pressures) or transferring patients 'up or down' to appropriate higher acuity, community or primary care settings.

This novel approach requires a new appreciation of knowledge that blends elements of emergency medicine, pre-hospital emergency medicine and primary care, the standards of which have now been set by bodies such as the Royal College of Surgeons of Edinburgh (with its Diploma in Urgent Medical Care) and UCLan (with its Masters programme in urgent medical care).

This is the first specialist book to bring the required knowledge to text. For those working in urgent medical care who seek a reference book, those preparing for the Royal College of Surgeons of Edinburgh examination, or those embarking on UCLan's Masters programme, this is your 'go to' literature.

Professor Stuart Maitland-Knibb
Director National Centre for Remote and
Rural Medicine

There is a perception that secondary care clinicians over-investigate, over-diagnose and over-treat while primary care equivalents struggle to manage the complexity of higher acuity conditions. While overstated, established training programmes and reference materials often do little to challenge or reverse these attitudes.

Increasing recognition is being given to the establishment of 'Urgent Medical Care' as a multidisciplinary subspecialty that offers a bridge between primary, secondary and community care, hence occupying an increasingly important 'space' in the establishment of emerging healthcare models. This novel approach offers real hope that solutions can be introduced to manage rising NHS demands.

This book aims to centralise guidance, research and material helpful for all clinicians working in urgent and unscheduled care (UUC) environments and to assist those preparing for the Royal College of Surgeons of Edinburgh's Diploma in Urgent Medical Care, the first formal examination of the emerging discipline.

Martin McGrath

ACKNOWLEDGEMENTS

For Caroline and Georgia, Mum and Dad, my hero Chris, Sue, Tom, Matt, Will, my other hero Uncle John, Auntie Sue, Joanna, Luke, Jonathan, Heather, Hayden, Olive, Maggie, Simon, Nicola, Pat, Tess, Anne, Matt, Mike, Luigi, Jo, Johnny, Kirstie, Lexie, Bea, Simon, Kim, John, Sarah, MGR and all our wonderful friends.

With special thanks to Stuart, Cathy, Nigel, Tricia, Caroline, Laura and Jo at UCLan and Alex and Taranpreet at Elsevier.

AMDG

SYMBOLS AND ABBREVIATIONS

A&E – Accident and Emergency
ACP – Advanced Community Practitioner
ANP – Advanced Nurse Practitioner
CCG – Clinical Commissioning Group
CQC – Care Quality Commission
CRM – Crew Resource Management
DoLS – Deprivation of Liberty Safeguards
DUMC – Diploma in Urgent Medical Care
E&D – Equality and Diversity
ECP – Emergency Care Practitioner
ED – Emergency Department
EMR – Electronic Medical Record
ENP – Emergency Nurse Practitioner
FFT – Friends and Family Test
FGM – Female Genital Mutilation
GCS – Glasgow Coma Scale
GMC – General Medical Committee
IAPT – Improved Access to Psychological Services
IMCA – Independent Mental Capacity Advocate
MCA – Mental Capacity Act
MDT – Multi-Disciplinary Team
MHA – Mental Health Act
MIMMS – Major Incident Medical Management and Support
NHSE – National Health Service England
OOH – Out of Hours
PHEM – Pre-Hospital Emergency Medicine
PPE – Personal Protective Equipment
PTSD – Post-Traumatic Stress Disorder
RCA – Root Cause Analysis
RCEM – Royal College of Emergency Medicine
RCGP – Royal College of General Practitioners
RCP – Royal College of Physicians
RCS(Ed) – Royal College of Surgeons of Edinburgh
SBAR – Situation, Background, Assessment, Recommendation
SDEC – Same Day Emergency Care
SEA – Significant Event Analysis
SRG – Systems Resilience Group
SUI – Serious Untoward Incident
TRiM – Trauma Risk Management
UCC – Urgent Care Centre
UEC – Urgent and Emergency Care
UTC – Urgent Treatment Centre
UUC – Urgent and Unscheduled Care

SECTION 1 ■ Recommended Doctor's Bag Contents – Adult

Indication	Drug
Mild to moderate pain	Paracetamol 500 mg tablets
	Ibuprofen 400 mg tablets
	Codeine 30 mg tablets
Severe pain	Diclofenac sodium 25 mg/mL 3 mL ampoules
	Diclofenac 100 mg suppositories
	Diamorphine 2.5–10 mg injection
Acute myocardial infarction and angina	Aspirin 300 mg tablets
	Glyceryl trinitrate 400 µg sublingual spray
Acute left ventricular failure	Furosemide 10 mg/mL injection
	Furosemide 40 mg tablets
Anaphylaxis	Adrenaline 1:1000 injection (1 mg/mL)
	Adrenaline 300 µg prefilled pen injection (important the user has been trained in its use)
	Chlorphenamine 10 mg/mL injection
	Hydrocortisone sodium succinate 100 mg injection
Asthma	Salbutamol 100 µg/dose metered-dose inhaler (MDI) with large volume spacer
	Prednisolone 5 mg tablets
Hypoglycaemia	Proprietary quick-acting carbohydrate (e.g. GlucoGel, Dextrogel)
	Glucagon 1 mg injection
	Glucose 20% injection 50 mL
Hypoadrenalism	Hydrocortisone sodium phosphate 100 mg/mL solution for injection
Suspected bacterial meningitis/meningococcal septicaemia	Benzyl penicillin 600 mg injection
	Cefotaxime 1 g injection
Nausea and vomiting	Cyclizine 50 mg/mL injection
	Metoclopramide 5 mg/mL injection
	Prochlorperazine 12.5 mg/mL injection
Opioid overdose	Naloxone 400 µg/mL injection
Seizures	Diazepam rectal solution 10 mg in 2.5 mL
	Midazolam oro-mucosal solution 5 mg/mL
Palliative care	Hyoscine butylbromide 20 mg/mL injection
	Midazolam 2 mg/mL injection
	Dexamethasone 2 mg tablets

Drugs for the doctor's bag: 1-adults. *Drug Ther Bull*. 2015;53(5):56. https://search.proquest.com/scholarly-journals/drugs-doctors-bag-1-adults/docview/1780555310/se-2?accountid=17233. doi: http://doi.org/10.1136/dtb.2015.5.0328.

SECTION 2 ■ Recommended Doctor's Bag Contents – Children

Indication	Drug
Acute pain	Paracetamol 120 mg/5 mL oral suspension Paracetamol 500 mg tablets Paracetamol 60 mg, 120 mg (or 125 mg), 250 mg suppositories Ibuprofen 100 mg/5 mL oral suspension Ibuprofen 200 mg tablets
Anaphylaxis	Adrenaline 1:1000 injection (1 mg/mL) Adrenaline 500 µg, 300 µg, 150 µg prefilled pen injection (it is important the user has been trained in its use) Chlorphenamine 10 mg/mL injection Hydrocortisone sodium succinate 100 mg injection
Respiratory conditions	Salbutamol 100 µg paediatric metered-dose inhaler (pMDI) via spacer (the patient may have their own spacer, or nebuliser) Dexamethasone 2 mg/5 mL oral solution Prednisolone 5 mg soluble tablets Salbutamol nebules 2.5 mg, 5 mg Ipratropium bromide nebules 250 µg/mL
Hypoglycaemia	Proprietary quick-acting carbohydrate (e.g. GlucoGel, Dextrogel) Glucagon 1 mg injection
Suspected bacterial meningitis/meningococcal septicaemia	Benzylpenicillin sodium 600 mg powder for injection Cefotaxime 1 g powder for solution for injection or infusion
Nausea and vomiting, gastroenteritis and dehydration	Oral rehydration salts
Opioid overdose	Naloxone 400 µg/mL injection
Seizures	Midazolam liquid oro-mucosal solution Diazepam 5 mg/2.5 mL, 10 mg/5 mL rectal tubes
Diluents	Water for injection Sodium chloride injection 0.9%

Drugs for the doctor's bag: 2-children. *Drug Ther Bull*. 2015;53(6):69. doi: http://doi.org/10.1136/dtb.2015.6.0334.

SECTION 3 ■ List of Notifiable Diseases

Notifiable Diseases

These diseases must be notified to local authority proper officers under the Health Protection (Notification) Regulations 2010

Acute encephalitis
Acute infectious hepatitis
Acute meningitis
Acute poliomyelitis
Anthrax
Botulism
Brucellosis
Cholera
COVID-19
Diphtheria
Enteric fever (typhoid or paratyphoid fever)
Food poisoning
Haemolytic uraemic syndrome (HUS)
Infectious bloody diarrhoea
Invasive group A streptococcal disease
Legionnaires' disease
Leprosy
Malaria
Measles
Meningococcal septicaemia
Mumps
Plague
Rabies
Rubella
Severe acute respiratory syndrome (SARS)
Scarlet fever
Smallpox
Tetanus
Tuberculosis
Typhus
Viral haemorrhagic fever (VHF)
Whooping cough
Yellow fever

Gov.uk Notifiable diseases and causative organisms: how to report. Available at: https://www.gov.uk/guidance/notifiable-diseases-and-causative-organisms-how-to-report. Accessed 28 December 2020.

Management

Working in Urgent Medical Care Systems

The Development of Urgent Care Systems – A Brief History

In 2009, the Primary Care Foundation noted the increasing need for primary care to address urgent care presentations in primary care[1] to:

- Avoid harm or distress to patient whose treatment or diagnosis may be delayed
- Relieve pressures on accident and emergency departments (A&Es) and avoidable admissions
- Improve patient experience of primary care
   The Health Foundation's 2018 report on emergency hospital admissions made the following observations[2]:
- One in three patients admitted to hospital in England as an emergency in 2015/16 had five or more health conditions, such as heart disease, stroke, type 2 diabetes, dehydration, hip fracture or dementia (up from 1 in 10 in 2006/07)
- The number of patients admitted urgently to hospital had increased by 42% over the past decade, far outstripping the total number of people who attended A&E departments, which was up by only 13%
- Patients arriving at A&E were sicker than ever before and more likely to need admission. This had grown for patients with multiple health conditions, as well as for older patients aged 85 or over, up by 58.9%
- Hospitals were treating patients more quickly, with overnight stays for those with five or more conditions lasting 10.8 nights in 2015/16 compared with 15.8 days a decade previously. The number of these patients admitted to hospital but discharged on the same day had increased by 373% over the same period

In 2020, NHSE set out its principles surrounding the structure of emergency and unscheduled care systems,[3] saying that:

- Urgent and emergency care (UEC) services perform a critical role in keeping the population healthy
- The National Health Service (NHS) responds to more than 110 million urgent calls or visits every year, so it is essential that the system works effectively
- Both UEC services play a specific part in supporting patients to receive the right care, by the right person, as quickly as possible. To help relieve pressure on A&E departments and to ensure patients get the right care, it is important to understand the difference between UEC:
  - Emergency: Life-threatening illnesses or accidents which require immediate, intensive treatment. Services that should be accessed in an emergency include ambulance (via 999) and emergency departments
  - Urgent: An illness or injury that requires urgent attention but is not a life-threatening situation. Urgent care services include a phone consultation through the NHS 111 Clinical Assessment Service, pharmacy advice, out-of-hours GP appointments and/or referral to an urgent treatment centre (UTC). If unsure what service is needed, NHS 111 can help to assess and direct to the appropriate services
- With increasing pressure on emergency services and as technology and the needs of the population change, the UEC system must also change to ensure a service fit for the future

The NHS separately established a National Elective and Emergency Care Directorate to:

- Provide national guidance and support to drive continuous improvement in elective and UEC services
- Work in partnership with other NHS organisations, system leaders, frontline staff, patients and key stakeholders (e.g. Royal colleges) to design, develop and implement best practice models of care that ensure patients see the right person, in the right place, as quickly as possible
- Establish the following workstreams:
  - Integrated urgent care
  - UTCs
  - Ambulance
  - Hospitals
  - Clinical review of NHS access standards
  - Reducing length of stay

Progress in transforming UEC services over recent years includes:

- 100% of the population of England are now able to access urgent care advice through the NHS 111 online service
- Development of the Integrated Urgent Care Service, so that more than half of the number of people calling NHS 111 now receive a clinical assessment and can be offered immediate advice or referred to the appropriate clinician for a face-to-face consultation
- Roll-out of UTCs across the country, providing a locally accessible and convenient service offering diagnosis and treatment of many of the most common reasons people attend A&E
- New standards for ambulance services to ensure that the sickest patients receive the fastest response and that all patients get the response they need first time
- National same day emergency care (SDEC) model for hospitals, building on existing ambulatory emergency care (AEC) efforts and reducing the number of patients admitted overnight for an emergency
- Establishment of an acute frailty programme to ensure the identification of frail patients within a few hours of their arrival to hospital and enable prompt, targeted management based on a comprehensive geriatric assessment approach

The NHS Long-Term Plan makes the following UEC services commitments:

- Providing a 24/7 urgent care service, accessible via NHS 111, which can provide medical advice remotely and, if necessary, refer directly to UTCs, GP (in and out of hours) and other community services (pharmacy, etc.), as well as ambulance and hospital services
- Implementing SDEC services across 100% of type 1 emergency departments, allowing for the rapid assessment, diagnosis and treatment of patients presenting with certain conditions and discharge home same day if clinically appropriate
- Focusing efforts to reduce the length of stay for patients in hospital longer than 21 days, reducing the risk of harm and providing care in the most clinically appropriate setting
- Working closely with primary and community care services to ensure an integrated, responsive healthcare service helping people stay well longer and receive preventative or primary treatment before it becomes an emergency

The Primary Care Foundation investigated seven myths of urgent care[4]:

Myth:
- Much of the care being delivered in A&E is primary care

Reality:
- The proportion of A&E cases that could be classified as primary care varies between 10% and 30%

Myth:
- There is always too much demand for services to cope with

Reality:
- It is rare for footfall to vary more than 50% from the daily average
- It should be possible to consistently deliver a timely one-stage response
- Inserting a triage or assessment stage in a bid to dispel queues and delays is wasteful of resources; the aim should be to match capacity to demand
- The reasons for queues developing can often be traced back to an understaffed unit due to absence, or clinicians working at different rates

Myth:
- Patients misuse urgent care services (the myth of inappropriate attenders)

Reality:
- There is a small group of users who consistently use the system in a different way from most, and many service plans are built around this minority group
- However, the majority of patients use the services appropriately, given the patients' perceived urgency at the time of use
- There is a tendency for services that do not have an effective operating model to blame the users rather than looking at their performance

Myth:
- It is important for commissioners to educate the public about services

Reality:
- There is some evidence that initiatives such as the expert patient programme and providing condition-specific information for patients are beneficial
- However, there is no evidence that general education about how to use a system has any impact
- For most people, using the urgent care system is a rare occurrence: once every 6 years for out-of-hours, on average every 3 years for A&E
- Giving information at the time of use does have an impact over time
- Such messaging needs reiterating consistently as a routine part of the consultation in all urgent care services over many years

Myth:
- It is safer for patients and better for service to triage everyone

Reality:

- There is good evidence that a rapid see and treat process is safer than a system involving multiple assessments and delays
- Triage is most often used to compensate for delays caused by poor capacity planning; there is no evidence that an assessment and triage service can improve utilisation and outcomes
- There is a danger that an assumption is made that the assessed patient is safe to wait when, in reality, the condition of some patients can change rapidly
- There is also a view that if everyone is assessed, patients can be directed to the most appropriate end point, but evidence suggests most patients will make the right choice themselves and if the service is available they will use it
- Evidence shows the feature patients value most is rapid access with minimal steps: they do not want multiple phone calls, ring back and delays, nor do they like to be assessed and then put to the back of a long queue in the waiting room

Myth:

- There is a direct link between A&E attendance and hospital admissions

Reality:

- There is some evidence that when A&E departments become overwhelmed junior staff will admit more people – the primary failure is in the A&E system not the volume presenting
- A number of key factors drive hospital admission numbers, including:
  - Number of individuals referred by GPs, 999, 111 and NHS Direct staff and out-of-hours services (which are all influenced by access to GP urgent care)
  - The efficiency of the process in A&E and acute medicine, including the availability of senior staff
- There is little or no evidence for the effectiveness of diversion schemes on admissions, and some cause serious safety concerns
- Good acute care by GPs in the community, combined with early assessment of the severity of an episode by the GP, has been shown to reduce admissions because there is time to arrange alternatives, keeping the patient away from hospital
- Out-of-hours providers should also focus on the clinical activity of their staff to ensure unnecessary referrals to hospital are avoided
- Targeted approaches, looking at each area where the decision to admit is made, such as improvements in AEC, are likely to be much more effective at reducing admissions

Myth:

- Commissioners should tender out-of-hours services frequently

Reality:

- Out-of-hours services are often put out to tender frequently, apparently with the view that this guarantees value for money
- Tender cycles which are too frequent make it difficult for a provider to invest, are expensive and may lead to too much focus on the tender price rather than quality, patient safety and the overall cost to the wider healthcare system

The Royal College of Emergency Medicine (RCEM) analysed A&E attendances, finding that[5]:

- Many patients attending A&E do so out of choice
- The greatest proportion of patients see A&E as the most appropriate place to attend with a healthcare problem they regard as urgent
- Nevertheless, a substantial proportion attended because they had been advised to do so by other healthcare providers. This suggests that, like patients, many healthcare providers behave and give advice based on a lack of confidence in viable alternatives to the A&E service

- In one-third of cases, patients had already received care from other healthcare providers for the same episode of illness – this demonstrates that there was also a lack of unplanned follow-up capacity for 30% of respondents who attended A&E

The Development of Urgent Care Systems – Challenges

The Care Quality Commission (CQC) report 'The state of care in urgent primary care services' inspected care delivered in urgent primary care services, such as walk-in and urgent care centres, NHS 111 and GP out-of-hours services,[6] finding that the very nature of urgent primary care services presents common challenges to providers, which then can adversely affect the quality of care, including:

- Staffing:
  - Staff can be dispersed over large areas and often work remotely, with little opportunity to build local teams among sessional and locum clinicians
  - They also work under pressure at times of high demand and unsocial hours, which affects recruitment and retention
  - Many UUC services experience very high turnover
- Commissioning:
  - Urgent care commissioning is complex
  - Contracts to provide a service in an area are often reprocured, and when an incumbent provider fails to win the tender, with a less experienced organisation taking over the contract, this leads to disruption, lost continuity and lost organisational memory and learning
  - Providers who are commissioned by a series of different geographically remote clinical commissioning groups (CCGs) may experience an adverse impact on the quality of service at some locations
- Resourcing: Sufficient resourcing to enable primary urgent care services to ease the pressure on acute hospitals
- Technology:
  - Used in more innovative ways that help to map capacity against demand in a local area and provide better communication between staff and other services, for example, using teleconferencing and other digital communication
  - Providing clinical support to develop existing staff, as well as designing pathways to deliver care that enables patients to stay out of hospital, with support in the community
- Integration:
  - Optimised so that demand from patients is balanced across the system, and the system can better respond to its local population in the right way at the right time
  - Important to allow people to benefit in both a health and social care setting
  - Includes areas such as the integrated Urgent Care Clinical Assessment Service, which brings together NHS 111 and GP out-of-hours services to provide 24/7 access to urgent care, clinical advice and treatment
  - Initiatives such as NHS England's work to embed pharmacy into the urgent care pathway by deploying prescribing pharmacists in integrated services
- Scale: Each year, the NHS provides approximately 110 million urgent same-day patient contacts. Approximately 85 million of these are urgent GP appointments, and the rest are emergency department (A&E) or minor injuries-type visits. Some estimates suggest that between 1.5 and 3 million people who visit an emergency department each year could have their needs addressed in other parts of the urgent care system
- Fluctuating and increasing demand: Demand for urgent services fluctuates dramatically throughout the year, with demand greatest over bank holidays and winter weekends

- Access to GP notes:
  - There is an inherently higher risk associated with urgent care services than with daytime general practice because a high percentage of patients present with acute illnesses such as sepsis. A high proportion of those using the services are also often more vulnerable, including those receiving end of life care
  - Urgent care is short and episodic and is most effective when services have access to people's medical records, as a minimum through the summary care record or local care record sharing services. It is also more effective for both clinicians and patients to have access to a person's primary care records from daytime general practice and information about their mental health and end of life care plans during 111 consultations. However, although information from the summary care record should readily be available, it is often difficult for clinicians to access
  - After using an urgent care service, information about the patient has traditionally been communicated back to their GP electronically and incorporated in their primary care record. Increasingly the most innovative local health economies are moving towards a more multiagency approach using online clinical systems that can record, share and use real-time patient information to provide better, more efficient integrated care

The Development of Urgent Care Systems – Evolving Solutions

Sir Bruce Keogh's Review of UEC[7] set out the plan for UEC networks to:
- Be based on the geographies required to give strategic oversight of UEC on a regional footprint
- Ensure that patients with more serious or life-threatening emergencies receive treatment in centres with the right facilities and expertise
- Ensure that individuals can have their urgent care needs met locally by services as close to home as possible
  System resilience groups (SRGs):
- Undertake operational leadership of local services
- Retain responsibility for ensuring the effective delivery of urgent care in their area, in coordination with an overall UEC strategy
  UEC networks:
- Operate strategically, covering a footprint of 1 to 5 million (depending on population density, rurality and local factors)
- Improve the consistency and quality of UEC by bringing together SRGs and other stakeholders to address challenges in the UEC system that are difficult for single SRGs to address in isolation
- Are involved in coordinating, integrating and overseeing care and setting shared objectives for the network where there is clear advantage in achieving commonality for delivery of efficient patient care (e.g. ambulance protocols, NHS 111 services, clinical decision support and access protocols to specialist services such as those for heart attack, stroke, major trauma, vascular surgery and critically ill children)
- Objectives for networks include:
  - Creating and agreeing an overarching, medium- to long-term plan
  - Designating urgent care facilities within the network
  - Setting and monitoring standards
  - Defining consistent pathways of care and equitable access to diagnostics and services for both physical and mental health
- Make arrangements to ensure effective patient flow through the whole urgent care system

- Maintain oversight and enable benchmarking of outcomes across the whole urgent care system
- Achieve resilience and efficiency in the urgent care system through coordination, consistency and economies of scale (e.g. agreeing common pathways and services across SRG boundaries)
- Coordinate workforce and training needs: establishing adequate workforce provision and sharing of resources
- Ensuring the building of trust and collaboration throughout the network
- Spread good and best practice

Networks should include within their boundary:
- Several SRGs
- Several CCGs
- All acute receiving hospitals and urgent care centres

UEC networks should ensure appropriate representation from key organisations that may include:
- Constituent SRGs
- Constituent CCGs (including lead commissioner for ambulance services)
- Receiving hospitals and urgent care centres
- Health and wellbeing board
- NHS 111 provider
- GP out-of-hours provider
- Ambulance service
- Community healthcare provider
- Mental health trust and provider
- Local authority
- NHS England regional representatives
- Community pharmacy services
- Health Education England
- Local Healthwatch

Alternative Urgent Care Models

Numerous systems around the world have been grappling with increasing UUC demand, for example:
- Australia, Denmark, France, Germany and the Netherland are[8]:
  - Expanding and increasingly centralising their urgent primary care
  - Concentrating emergency care provision at fewer hospitals
  - Improving coordination between urgent primary care and emergency care
  - Designing their payment systems to support these reforms
  - Recognising challenges that include emergency department (ED) overcrowding, long waiting times and increasing numbers of ED visits
- Ireland uses variations of UUC provision across different regions[9]

The Evolution of Urgent Care Workforces

GPs and emergency nurse practitioners (ENPs) were traditionally groups that did not work alongside each other within ED/UCCs. A study looking at the evolving GP-led UCC model in which both ENPs and GPs were able to request investigations found[10]:
- GPs working within an ED setting adjusted their role to fit the demands of both the patient and the wider healthcare system

- Eight key factors appeared to have facilitated the development of this team: appointment of leaders, perception of fair workload, education on roles/skill sets and development of these, shared professional understanding, interdisciplinary working, ED collaboration, clinical guidelines and social

Patient Choice and Behaviour

Studies undertaken before the advent of specific UUC models into why patients sought UEC often focused on 'utilisation' behaviour for specific conditions (e.g. mental health, long-term conditions) or other 'imposed' organisational factors.[11]

Newer studies looking at patient interaction with UUC systems have noted that these systems have evolved as a response to health 'consumerism', rhetoric of 'patient choice' and the aspiration to use urgent care to divert people away from overcrowded emergency services.

Research about help-seeking for urgent and/or emergency care showed that:

- People seek urgent care about symptoms that they perceive to be severe, unusual or worsening or causing pain
- Users make contact for medical care and advice and to seek reassurance
- Although help-seeking is influenced by previous experiences and perceptions of accessibility, several studies suggest that people often just do not know where to go and go through a mental process of considering and eliminating uncertain options (e.g. people may use emergency department services when general practice is not available, to access more 'specialist' care or because the emergency department offers shorter waiting times and ease of access)
- Patients increasingly using online information to shape decision making

The theoretical background of health service utilisation is complex:

- Different theories include variations in cognition, decision making and learning and individual beliefs as triggers to help-seeking
- The 'Health Belief Model' describes psychological and motivational determinants of health service use, where cues to action (e.g. pain) and the readiness to act are modified by individual and demographic characteristics such as gender, personality and social class
- Some studies show that service use is influenced by individual level predisposing factors (e.g. health beliefs, age, education, social position) but also by community and enabling resources (e.g. income, access to transport)

Newer studies attempt to refocus attention on the 'work' people do to make sense of urgent care and categorise this into three main areas:

- 'Illness work' suggests that:
  - People make sense of illness by interpreting the severity of symptoms, managing physical and psychological state, assessing risks and making decisions about accessing services
  - Symptoms that are sudden, unusual or 'serious' or that interfere with daily life (e.g. impaired mobility) are likely to prompt help-seeking
  - Uncertainty about symptoms often provoke anxiety
  - Those reporting lower levels of anxiety tend to seek reassurance from urgent care services such as NHS 111, but those who are more worried use emergency care
  - Patients seek reassurance from health professionals or members of lay networks to 'be on the safe side' and manage potential risks
  - Younger and East European patients are more likely to use NHS 111 as a first port of call
  - Many consider the perceived limitations of their own expertise when interpreting and managing symptoms and so draw on others in their social network to sanction decisions (e.g. asking others about whether to contact a particular health service)

- Those who feel responsible for the health of others (children or a partner) and where the frequency of interaction is high (e.g. living in the same household) are highly influenced by social networks when deciding to use the UUC service
- 'Moral work' suggests that:
  - Patients undertake work to present as an appropriate, legitimate or responsible user of healthcare – 'a credible patient'[12]
  - There may be a tension between a patient's desire to represent themselves as responsible (i.e. not a 'time waster') and the desire to delegate illness work to healthcare professionals
  - 'Moral work' is multifaceted, undertaking the moral responsibility of being a 'good self-manager' (taking responsibility for own health, and using knowledge to manage risks) to enable 'appropriate' judgements about the nature of urgent symptoms; patients weigh up the risk of harm against taking action[13]
  - These patients are keen to demonstrate their responsibility, providing accounts of when they had not sought help or examples of symptoms they considered trivial; they describe themselves as 'copers' who tolerate symptoms and perform self-care as much as possible
  - Patients make efforts to compare and reference service use against that of 'others', sometimes using social networks to sanction help-seeking and alleviate individual responsibility for decision making
  - Patients can cite others (parents, managers, etc.) as the reason they seek help
- 'Navigation work' suggests that:
  - Patients identify and make sense of the range of services on offer and how to access healthcare services
  - Patients make choices between what is available (e.g. staffing, resources, technology), accessible (the ease with which a health service can be physically reached) and 'accommodating' (e.g. convenient opening hours)
  - Patients may attend A&E because it offers a 'one stop shop' where additional specialist facilities (e.g. x-ray) can be accessed, thereby avoiding a potentially wasted journey elsewhere, or otherwise use an urgent care centre because it is considered more 'pleasant'
  - Patients base decisions more on efficiency and convenience rather than an assessment of severity or clinical need

  Taking the population as a whole:
- Service users hold strong moral views and are highly sensitive to arguments about 'inappropriate' help-seeking in the emergency department
- However, patients often externalise these judgements such that moral rules are applied to others (e.g. characterising others as 'time wasters')[14–16]
- Patients make choices mainly based on what is accessible at a given time of day, geographic and transport accessibility and social or peer advice

  The relevance of this is:
- The interaction between thinking (sense-making) and action (help-seeking)
- That patients use their social networks work to interpret illness, make moral judgements and navigate services
- UUC system designers should focus less on blaming 'incorrect' sense-making and 'inappropriate' decision making, and begin to support patient decision making
- Advertising and health education campaigns should better reflect the social and temporal (time of day) drivers that might push people towards particular services

UUC Operational Environments

NHSE's principles surrounding the structure of emergency and unscheduled care systems describe the difference between emergency and urgent care as[17]:

- Emergency: 'Life-threatening illnesses or accidents which require immediate, intensive treatment. Services that should be accessed in an emergency include ambulance (via 999) and emergency departments'
- Urgent: 'An illness or injury that requires urgent attention but is not a life-threatening situation. Urgent care services include a phone consultation through the NHS 111 Clinical Assessment Service, pharmacy advice, out-of-hours GP appointments, and/or referral to an UTC. If unsure what service is needed, NHS 111 can help to assess and direct to the appropriate service/s'

Urgent and unscheduled care can therefore be delivered in a number of different environments that include

- Primary care
- Hospitals – including in emergency departments
- UTCs
- Urgent care centres
- Walk-in clinics
- The community – district nursing, etc.
- NHS 111
- Home visiting services
- Roadside/'prehospital' – ambulance services

The CQC describes urgent care centres as follows[18]:

- Most urgent care centres are based in the community, either in stand-alone premises or colocated with other services such as GP out-of-hours services
- Some are located on a hospital site but are run by a provider organisation that is not the hospital itself. Despite being run by different organisations, urgent care centres on a hospital site usually work closely with the hospital's emergency department, which may stream patients to the urgent care centre after assessing them for suitability and redirecting them
- Urgent care centres are commissioned by CCGs
- Some providers run only one or two urgent care centres, whereas others are large organisations that may also provide other types of services, such as GP out-of-hours services
- Many of these larger organisations hold contracts across England and have centralised governance for their services, which are coordinated locally by service managers and senior clinicians
- Clinicians may be directly employed, self-employed contractors or a mixture of both. Urgent care and walk-in centres also regularly use locums as well as staff employed through a contract. Many contracted staff may also carry out their duties for the same provider from more than one of its registered locations.

NHS 111 Services

NHS 111 provides access to both treatment and clinical advice with the following principles:

- Established in 2012 to replace NHS Direct as a free, urgent but nonemergency number to work alongside 999
- Available 24 hours a day, 365 days a year
- Covers England, Scotland and parts of Wales but with services delivered by different providers in different geographic areas, each commissioned by the local CCG
- By integrating technology, calls can be directed to services around the country to enable available resources to handle demand when national contingency plans are invoked
- The NHS 111 directory of services (DOS) enables calls to be directed to the most appropriate and locally available service
- A number of these services are provided as part of wider out-of-hours services or urgent care services by the same provider
- Some 111 services are commissioned by a CCG and delivered by an independent provider, whereas some providers are social enterprises that reinvest any profits back into services

rather than passing them on to shareholders as some other 111 providers do. Others are provided by ambulance services
- Calls to the 111 number are directed to the local 111 provider. They are answered by a nonclinical call handler who is trained to use a computer decision support system called NHS Pathways to manage calls
- NHS Pathways is a nationally validated algorithm built on clinical expertise combined with a real-time DOS available for patients, which identifies the best source of help for the caller; this may be to speak to a clinician working for NHS 111, to attend another service, such as the patient's own GP, or to self-care
- In emergencies, the call handler will arrange a 999 ambulance transfer to an emergency department, where necessary

GP Out-of-Hours Services

Following points are applicable to Out-of-hours services:
- They provide urgent primary care when GP surgeries are closed
- They usually provide face-to-face consultations in primary care centres, home visits and telephone consultations
- Most patients are directed to these services by NHS 111 or, in some cases, emergency departments
- Some primary care centres accept walk-in patients, while others require patients to have called NHS 111 before they arrive
- They use nurses, advanced nurse practitioners, pharmacists and paramedics, as well as GPs
- Typically, most out-of-hours GPs are self-employed sessional contractors, whereas the other clinicians may be directly employed or contractors
- Some services use a high number of agency staff

Working in Multidisciplinary Teams

Multidisciplinary teams (MDTs) are teams of professionals from different disciplines in primary, community, social care and mental-health services who work together to plan a patient's care.[19] There is no one set form of how MDTs must be organised. The level of integration can range from a single professional with continued responsibility for care drawing on other staff or services for input, through to multiple professionals holding shared responsibility for care of the service user, potentially drawing on a much wider pool of services and professionals.

The RCP issued guidance surrounding medical teams[20]:
- Indicating that success depended on:
  - Common sense of purpose
  - Clear understanding of objectives
  - Resources to achieve objectives
  - Mutual respect among team members
  - Values members' strengths and weaknesses
  - Mutual trust
  - Willingness to speak openly
  - Range of skills to deal effectively with tasks
  - Range of personal styles for team roles
- Advising that:
  - All healthcare professionals need to be aware of the benefits of effective team working (i.e. increased performance, productivity, patient satisfaction, clinical outcomes and staff morale)
  - There should be an increased focus in clinical environments on goal setting
  - Goals should be agreed at all team meetings, including shift handovers

- Teams should be proactive at formulating objectives around personal performance, team development and education activities
- Roles and responsibilities should be explicitly stated at the start of all team activities. There should not be a reliance on hierarchy and status quo to identify these responsibilities
- Medical professionals should be trained in the supportive context of a multiprofessional team
- Recommending the following checklist:
  - Are team members clear about what we are trying to achieve?
  - Can we rely on one another? Do we work supportively to get the job done?
  - Do we have lively debates about how best to work?
  - Do we meet sufficiently often to ensure effective communication and cooperation?
  - Are people in the team quick to offer help and find new ways of doing things?
  - Do we all have influence on final decisions?
  - Are we careful to keep each other informed about work issues?
  - Is there a feeling of trust and safety in this team?
  - Are we enthusiastic about innovation?
  - Are team members committed to achieving the set objectives?
  - Can we safely discuss errors and mistakes?
  - Is there is a climate of constructive criticism in this team?

999 Call Handling and Dispatch

Ambulance services are at the heart of the UEC system. The NHS plan includes changes to ambulance standards so that by 2021 all ambulance services will:

- Meet all targets and deliver all patient outcomes
- Be efficient and effective
- Have a satisfied, happy and productive workforce
- Be integrated into the wider Urgent & Emergency Care System
- Be digitally fit for the future
- Aim to treat patients by skilled paramedics in their own home, given advice over the telephone or taken to a more appropriate setting outside hospital

Future plans include:

- Delivering a safe reduction in ambulance conveyance, which means that patients are taken to hospital only if that is the right place for them
- Making sure that no one arriving by ambulance should wait more than 30 minutes from arrival to handover to a clinician at hospital
- Supporting ambulance services to meet response time standards, as set out in the ambulance quality indicators
- Developing an ambulance data set to better understand and support improved delivery of patient care, and identify opportunities for system improvement

The Characteristics of Good and Bad Urgent Care Services

The CQC inspects services under five main categories but has found that the following characteristics are relevant in providers of good and outstanding UUC care[6]:

Effective communication with staff. These providers:

- Develop processes to communicate effectively with staff, despite the workforce being dispersed across different areas and locations
- Provide appropriate clinical supervision and support for their staff (e.g. NHS 111 providers enabling call handlers to get clinical advice quickly, often using methods that were

simple but effective, such as the call handlers holding up signs to attract the clinicians' attention)

- Share learning from significant events, audits and complaints effectively across the team
- Identify effective ways to communicate these with their staff, such as newsletters and screensaver alerts which are used regularly
- Have effective two-way communication between frontline staff and managers, with staff saying that managers were approachable and supportive
- Pay close attention to communication between call-handlers and clinicians, ensuring that call-handlers could access clinical guidance quickly and consistently
- Have well-established systems for monitoring the quality of their performance and for supporting call-handlers or clinicians if there are concerns about quality
Initial assessment of patients. These providers:
- Ensure they give a timely initial assessment to patients, typically either using a healthcare assistant working with clinical supervision from a nurse or GP, or by training reception staff to use an assessment system validated as safe for (trained) nonclinicians to use, such as NHS Pathways
Responsive to the population. These providers:
- Respond well to their local population, including engaging with patients and tailoring their services to their population's needs
- Use all feedback constructively, including feedback from significant events, complaints and surveys
- Analyse this information to identify trends and take action to address problems
- Can demonstrate how they use feedback from patients to improve services
- Are proactive in developing a clear understanding of the health and social care needs of particular populations such as people receiving end of life care or those with chronic illness
Recruiting staff. These providers:
- Tackle the difficulty in recruiting GPs to work in this sector, including turning to a multidisciplinary model
- Embed this with appropriate clinical supervision and a clear understanding of the competencies of the individuals in the service, with any changes to patient pathways ensuring that patients are seen by the most appropriate professional in a timely way
Cooperating with the wider health and social care system. These providers:
- Acknowledge that the UEC sector as a whole is becoming more integrated with other providers (e.g. where contracts are split between organisations, one of whom may deliver the out-of-hours component and another the 111 service, but with the expectation that both services work together)
- Are able to demonstrate effective joint working with other providers, even where there was no formal integration by way of contracts
- Demonstrate a proactive approach to working with other providers at operational level
Governance. These providers:
- Have a well-developed and independent system of audit and use innovative tools to monitor the quality of care
- Use peer review and external audit, including that offered by Urgent Health UK (a membership organisation for social enterprise urgent care providers)
- Submit themselves to an external audit and commit to peer review of serious incidents
In contrast, the following characteristics are relevant in providers who offer inadequate care or need improvement[6]:
Initial assessment of patients. These providers:
- Fail to perform a reliable and timely initial assessment of patients to identify those needing urgent care (mainly involves services providing face-to-face assessments, such as primary care centres run by GP out-of-hours services and urgent care centres)

- Fail to deliver prompt definitive care to these patients, once identified (mainly involves GP out-of-hours services, especially the home visiting element)
- Deliver on routine urgency target home visits but fail to meet their target for the smaller number of patients assessed as needing an urgent home visit
- Have an unreliable form of initial assessment if the patient has to wait more than 15 minutes for a definitive clinical assessment

Poor leadership. These providers:

- Provide poor leadership which in turn affects the whole service with knock on effects on staff turnover and recruitment
- Experience a wide range in the quality of services across the country delivered by the same provider – often as a result of a disconnect between management and oversight at national and local level
- Create a sense of isolation, being a small part of a large organisation, with a marked gap between central management and front-line staff and a failure to apply learning from one part of the organisation to another
- Have an unresponsive and unsupportive leadership which inhibits good local work
- Have a blame culture when things went wrong

Weak systems and formal processes. These providers:

- Are unable to provide evidence to demonstrate that their processes are sufficiently robust to meet the demands of providing urgent care
- May have policies and systems in place but fail to clearly define and embed them
- Fail to identify all incidents and ensure that learning and outcomes are effectively shared to prevent the same thing happening again

Governance. These providers:

- Fail to audit cases and take action on the basis of poor performance
- Tolerate the attitude that 'it's better to have a bad doctor than no doctor'
- Do not have robust processes for managing safeguarding referrals or for passing on safeguarding concerns to a patient's registered GP

Recruitment, staffing and workforce planning. These providers:

- Operate with low levels of staff
- Do not have reliable processes for minimising risk and maximising efficiency when there are not enough staff
- Do not empower their staff to make operational decisions
- Have high rates of self-employed clinical staff
- Do not deal with peak in demand
- Recruit 'inappropriate' staff to fill gaps with insufficient competencies
- Do not provide adequate supervision and support or adjusting pathways if clinicians did not have competencies or up-to-date skills and knowledge

Poor communication. These providers:

- Have inadequate systems to communicate with their clinicians
- Do not address the challenges of a dispersed workforce
- Lack information to show that learning is being disseminated
- Do not have effective systems to act on alerts issued by the Medicines and Healthcare products Regulatory Agency about medicines
- Do not ensure that NICE (National Institute for Health and Care Excellence) guidelines and updates are received and acted on in a timely way

Poor medicines management. These providers:

- Have varying standards of stocking, monitoring and availability of drugs
- Have limited access to controlled drugs
- Store drugs centrally but then have no one available to collect them and take them to the patient

Impact of commissioning arrangements. These providers:

- Lack sufficient funding from commissioners to deliver a high-quality service
- Provide services across multiple areas with variations that include differing service specifications and funding between CCGs, which prevent them from achieving economies of scale in how they deliver the service
- Are constrained by limits placed by some commissioners that mean they cannot adapt their services to local needs (e.g. moving to a more multidisciplinary model to support staffing)

Providing Support to Urgent Care Staff

There is increasing evidence of a need to support the clinical workforce in general. The General Medical Council (GMC) has established the need to consider support for doctors, stating[21]:

- The wellbeing of doctors is vital because there is abundant evidence that workplace stress in healthcare organisations affects quality of care for patients as well as doctors' own health
- In two studies, researchers found that doctors with high levels of burnout had between 45% and 63% higher odds of making a major medical error in the following 3 months, compared with those who had low levels
- Patient satisfaction is also markedly higher in healthcare organisations and teams where staff health and wellbeing are better
- The wellbeing of doctors is linked to a significant problem with retaining doctors, which is exacerbating existing difficulties with providing the numbers of doctors needed to support our health services
- Just under half of doctors working in hospitals and other secondary care organisations in England are considering leaving the organisations in which they work
- Nearly one in five doctors (17%) are considering leaving the NHS altogether
- The eighth National GP Worklife Survey in England, published in 2017, reported the lowest levels of job satisfaction among GPs and revealed the highest levels of stress since the survey began in 1998; it also showed that 35% of GPs were intending to quit direct patient care within the next 5 years
- More than a third of doctors working in secondary care also indicated that they had been unwell as a result of work-related stress in the previous year (37% of doctors in the 2018 NHS Staff Survey in England)
- Nearly one in four doctors in training in the United Kingdom and one in five trainers said they felt burnt out to a high or very high degree because of their work (2018, GMC national training surveys (NTS))
- Nearly half of doctors in training reported working beyond their rostered hours, while one in five said that their working pattern had left them short of sleep
- Doctors working in emergency medicine, where crisis management has become the norm, are amongst those experiencing the highest levels of burnout. The 2019 NTS revealed that doctors working in emergency medicine had very high rates of burnout (69.2% of trainees and 63% of trainers reported moderate or high levels of burnout). This is considerably higher than the average (49.9% of doctors in training overall and 46.8% of trainers)

Supporting Workers After Traumatic Events

Those working in UUC environments are likely to be involved at some time in a traumatic event. There is mixed evidence surrounding the usefulness of individual debriefs/counselling after involvement in traumatic events:

- Some studies show that offering critical incident stress debrief (CISD; developed as a therapeutic technique to be used with first responders after exposure to an excessively stressful or horrific critical incident) is associated with significantly less alcohol use and significantly greater quality of life post intervention, with no significant effects on posttraumatic stress or psychological distress.[22]
- Other studies suggest that research on CISD does not support its continued use[23]
- The military has developed Trauma Risk Management (TRiM) as a trauma-focused peer support system designed to help people who have experienced a traumatic, or potentially traumatic, event. TRiM practitioners are nonmedical personnel who have undergone specific training allowing them to understand the effects that traumatic events can have upon people.[24]

References

1. Primary Care Foundation. http://www.primarycarefoundation.co.uk/urgent-care-in-general-practice. html. Accessed 24 May 2020.
2. The Health Foundation. Emergency hospital admissions in England: which may be avoidable and how? https://www.health.org.uk/publications/emergency-hospital-admissions-in-england-which-may-be-avoidable-and-how. Accessed 24 May 2020.
3. NHSE. About urgent and emergency care. https://www.england.nhs.uk/urgent-emergency-care/about-uec/. Accessed 24 May 2020.
4. The Primary Care Foundation. The 7 myths of urgent care. https://www.primarycarefoundation.co.uk/the-7-myths-of-urgent-care.html. Accessed 24 May 2020.
5. Royal College of Emergency Medicine. Time to act – urgent care and A&E: the patient perspective. https://www.health.org.uk/publications/emergency-hospital-admissions-in-england-which-may-be-avoidable-and-how. Accessed 24 May 2020.
6. Care Quality Commission. The state of care in urgent primary care services. https://www.cqc.org.uk/sites/default/files/20180619%20State%20of%20care%20in%20urgent%20primary%20care%20services. pdf. Accessed 24 May 2020.
7. NHS England. Role and establishment of urgent and emergency care networks. https://www.nhs.uk/NHSEngland/keogh-review/Documents/Role-Networks-advice-RDs%201.1FV.pdf. Accessed 24 May 2020.
8. Baier N, Geissler S, Bech M, et al. Emergency and urgent care systems in Australia, Denmark, England, France, Germany and the Netherlands – analyzing organization, payment and reforms. *Health Policy.* 2019;123(1):1–10. https://doi.org/10.1016/j.healthpol.2018.11.001.
9. Foley C, Droog E, Boyce M, et al. *Patient Experience of Different Regional Models of Urgent and Emergency Care: A Cross-Sectional Survey Study.* British Medical Journal Publishing Group; 2017.
10. Morton S, Igantowicz A, Gnani S, et al. *Describing Team Development Within a Novel GP-Led Urgent Care Centre Model: A Qualitative Study.* British Medical Journal Publishing Group; 2016.
11. Turnbull J, Pope C, Prichard J, et al. A conceptual model of urgent care sense-making and help-seeking: a qualitative interview study of urgent care users in England. *BMC Health Serv Res.* 2019;19(1). https://doi.org/10.1186/s12913-019-4332-6.
12. Adamson J, Ben-Shlomo Y, Chaturvedi N, et al. Exploring the impact of patient views on 'appropriate' use of services and help seeking: a mixed method study. *Br J Gen Pract.* 2009;59(564):226. https://doi.org/10.3399/bjgp09X453530.
13. Ellis J, Boger E, Latter S, et al. Conceptualisation of the 'good' self-manager: a qualitative investigation of stakeholder views on the self-management of long-term health conditions. *Soc Sci Med.* 2017;176:25–33. https://doi.org/10.1016/j.socscimed.2017.01.018.

14. Goode J, Hanlon G, Luff D, et al. Male vallers to NHS direct: the assertive carer, the new dad and the reluctant patient. *Health*. 2004;8(3):311–328. https://doi.org/10.1177/1363459304043468.
15. Houston AM, Pickering AJ. Do I don't I call the doctor: a qualitative study of parental perceptions of calling the GP out-of-hours. *Health Expect*. 2000;3(4):234–242. https://doi.org/10.1046/j.1369-6513.2000.00109.x.
16. Jackson CJ, Dixon-Woods M, Hsu R, et al. A qualitative study of choosing and using an NHS Walk-in Centre. *Fam Pract*. 2005;22(3):269–274. https://doi.org/10.1093/fampra/cmi018.
17. NHSE. About urgent and emergency care. https://www.england.nhs.uk/urgent-emergency-care/about-uec/. Accessed 24 May 2020.
18. Care Quality Commission. The state of care in independent online primary health services: findings from CQC's programme of comprehensive inspections in England. https://www.cqc.org.uk/sites/default/files/20180322_state-of-care-independent-online-primary-health-services.pdf. Accessed 24 May 2020.
19. NHSE. MDT Development – Working Toward an Effective Multidisciplinary/Multiagency Team. https://www.england.nhs.uk/wp-content/uploads/2015/01/mdt-dev-guid-flat-fin.pdf. Accessed 24 May 2020.
20. Royal College of Physicians. Improving teams in healthcare. https://www.rcplondon.ac.uk/projects/improving-teams-healthcare. Accessed 24 May 2020.
21. General Medical Council. Caring for Doctors Caring for Patients. https://www.gmc-uk.org/-/media/documents/caring-for-doctors-caring-for-patients_pdf-80706341.pdf. Accessed 24 May 2020.
22. Tuckey MR, Scott JE. Group critical incident stress debriefing with emergency services personnel: a randomized controlled trial. *Anxiety Stress Coping*. 2014;27(1):38–54. https://doi.org/10.1080/10615806.2013.809421.
23. Burchill C. Critical incident stress debriefing: helpful, harmful, or neither? *J Emerg Nurs*. 2019;45(6):611–612. https://doi.org/10.1016/j.jen.2019.08.006.
24. Greenberg N, Langston V, Jones N. *Trauma Risk Management (TRiM) in the UK Armed Forces*. British Medical Journal Publishing Group; 2008.

Using Technology in Urgent Medical Care

Definitions and Meanings

DIGITAL TECHNOLOGY

Innovation based on the binary computing system, which enables huge amounts of information to be compressed on small storage devices, preserved and transported or transmitted – this has led to a transformation in how societies communicate, learn and work.

DIGITAL HEALTH

The convergence of digital technologies with health, healthcare, living and society to enhance the efficiency of healthcare delivery – better understood as 'health connectivity', which involves the use of information and communication technologies to help address health problems and challenges. Figure 2.1 illustrates a digital health 'ecosystem' within healthcare. It encompasses sub-sectors such as:
- e Health
- m-Health
- Tele-health
- Health information technology (IT)
- Telemedicine[1]

HEALTH TECHNOLOGY

The application of organised knowledge and skills that are developed to solve a health problem and improve quality of lives[2] in the form of:
- Devices

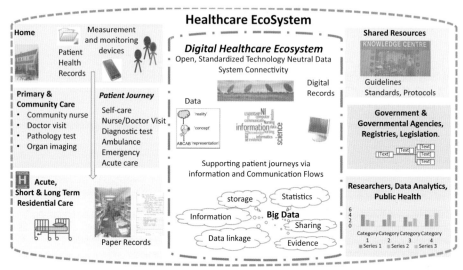

Fig. 2.1   Interconnectivity: A digital health 'ecosystem' within healthcare. (From Hovenga and Lowe, 2020.)

- Medicines
- Vaccines
- Procedures
- Systems

So, urgent care technology describes 'digital health' in the 'urgent and unscheduled care' environment and includes:

- Medical record systems
- Monitoring
- Near-patient investigations
- Radiology
- Remote consulting/interactions – 'Telehealth'
- Data analytics

Drivers for Change – Overview

Recognised drivers for the increasing use of technology in urgent care include:

- System
  - Efficiencies and productivity
  - Patient outcomes
  - Workforce challenges
  - Best practice
  - Evidence base
- Individual
  - Patient preference
  - 'Acceptability' of technology

- Commercial
  - Cost
  - Patient outcomes

Drivers for Change – System

One of the best examples of a 'system' drive for change is the National Health Service (NHS) Long Term Plan,[3] which promotes the use of technology to ease pressures associated with:
- Funding
- Workforce
- Strain in primary care and acute services
  The Plan identifies several practical steps that have direct relevance to UUC provision, including:
- Boost 'out-of-hospital' care
- Redesign and reduce pressure on emergency hospital services
- Give patients more control over their own health and more personalised care when they need it
- Digitally enable primary and outpatient care across the NHS
- Increase focus by local NHS organisations on population health
  The NHS Digital Toolkit[4] has been subsequently generated specifically to offer:
- Straight-forward digital access
- Access to records and care plans anywhere
- Decision support and artificial intelligence (AI)
- Predictive techniques to support local health systems to plan care for populations
- Intuitive tools to capture data as a by-product of care
- Privacy protection and patient control over their medical record
- Increased focus on population health
- Linked clinical, genomic and other data to support the development of new treatments
- Mandated and rigorously enforced tech standards
- World-leading health IT industry
- Redesigned emergency hospital services
- More control over own health and more personalised care
- Digitally enabled primary and outpatient care

Drivers for Change – Individual

There is arguably an increase in 'consumerism in healthcare', with research[5] showing that a patient's satisfaction of a clinical encounter relates to:
- Transparency (67%)
- Wait time/speed of appointment booking (64%)
- Convenience of waiting time (62%)
- Convenience of location or channel (60%)
- Responsiveness of follow-up after appointment (51%)
- Whether the doctor prescribes what is wanted (46%)
  Even before the advent of covid-related changes, the same study shows that ever-increasing numbers of patients would consider using:
- Walk-in/retail clinics

- Virtual care/digital therapeutics
- On-demand healthcare services

Surveys also show a huge global increase in 'connectivity' and the ability of patients to use technology to access healthcare.[6] Around the world:

- 56% are urbanised
- 67% are mobile users
- 57% are internet users
- 45% are social media users
- 42% are mobile social media users

Future Technology

Digital health is an emerging capability that will undoubtedly expand considerably. Its ability to further operate at scale depends upon[1]:

- Creation of a robust health IT infrastructure for storage, access to health data and information sharing
- Implementation of accessible electronic health records (EHRs) and investment in basic digital technologies that accelerate digitalisation
- Addressing the challenge of interoperability
- Establishing a robust governance framework to support a culture of digital transformation
- Developing digital leadership skills and improving the digital literacy of staff and patients

Relevance of Health Technology in UUC Settings

Technology that is less relevant to urgent care includes:

- Telehealth
  - Long-term condition monitoring
- Telecare
  - Activity/fall monitoring
  - Remote medication management
- Mobile health
  - Wearables
  - Wellness and fitness apps
- Health analytics
  - Genomics
  - Precision medicine

Technology that is more relevant to urgent care includes:

- Telehealth
  - Video/telephone consultations
- Mobile health
  - Medical apps and texts
- Health analytics
  - Data analytics
- Digitised health systems

- Patient-held medical records
- Provider-held medical records
- Near-patient testing
  - Radiological
  - Monitoring
  - Laboratory investigations

Urgent Treatment Centres

NHSE's 'Urgent Treatment Centres – Principles and Standards' 2017 set out[7] that an urgent treatment centre should offer:

- A consistent route to access urgent appointments booked through NHS 111, ambulance services and general practice
- The expectation of reduced attendance at, and conveyance to, accident and emergency (A&E)
- Protocols to manage critically ill and injured adults and children who arrive unexpectedly
- Access to investigations including swabs, pregnancy tests and urine dipsticks and culture
- Near patient blood testing, such as glucose, haemoglobin, D-dimer and electrolytes
- Electrocardiograms (ECG) and, in some urgent treatment centres, near-patient troponin testing
- Bedside diagnostics and plain x-ray facilities, particularly of the chest and limbs (desirable and considerably increase the assessment capability of an urgent treatment centre, particularly where not co-located with A&E)
- E-prescribing
- Arrangements for staff to access an up-to-date electronic patient care record (SCR or local equivalent)
- Systems interoperability that makes use of nationally-defined interoperability and data standards
- The ability to make capacity and wait time data available to the local health economy close to real-time

In this sense, a 'standard' technology offering that offers a real opportunity to minimise hospital attendances and admissions includes:

- Radiology
  - X-ray
  - Ultrasound (FAST [focused assessment using sonography for trauma] scanning)
  - Bladder scanning
- Laboratory
  - Urinalysis/pregnancy testing
  - Near-patient blood testing
    - FBC, U&E, LFT, amylase
    - VBG/ABG, troponin, D-dimer
- Medical records system
  - Integration/remote bookings
  - Full electronic medical record (EMR)/summary care record (SCR)

NHS Urgent Treatment Centres are based on class-leading Urgent Care Centres such as this one in Corby (illustrated in Figs 2.2 to 2.7).

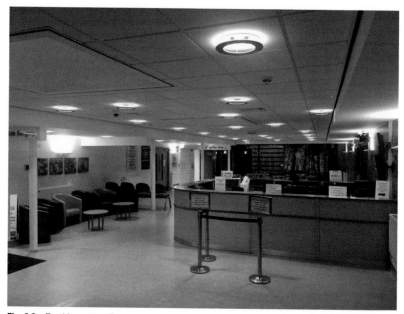

Fig. 2.2 Booking area: Easy-access reception with open waiting area before patients enter triage rooms.

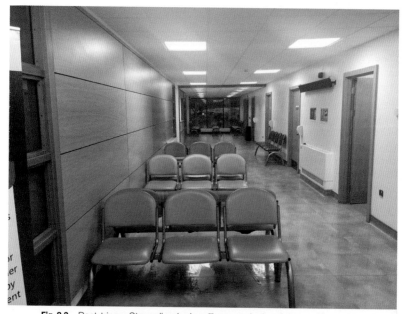

Fig. 2.3 Post-triage: Streamlined minor illness and minor injury waiting areas.

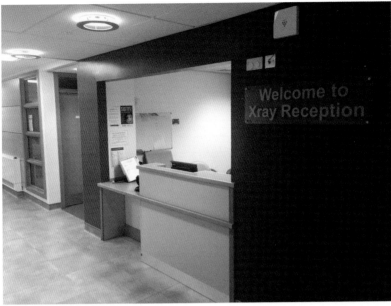

Fig. 2.4 Radiology: On-site X-ray and ultrasound facility plus plaster room.

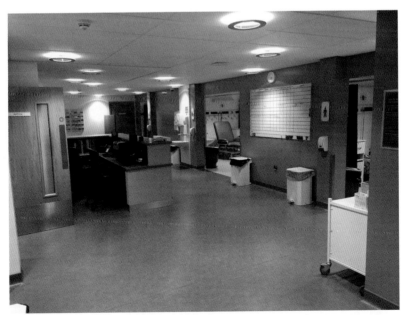

Fig. 2.5 Observation bay: Separate male, female and child areas to allow the assessment, treatment and monitoring of high acuity patients.

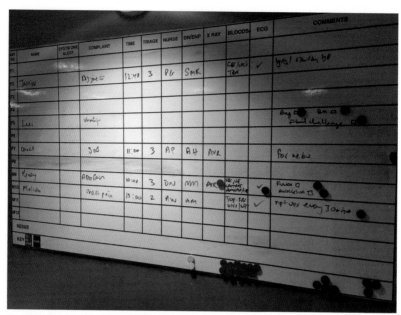

Fig. 2.6 Organisation: Coordination of team-based assessment, treatment and monitoring activities.

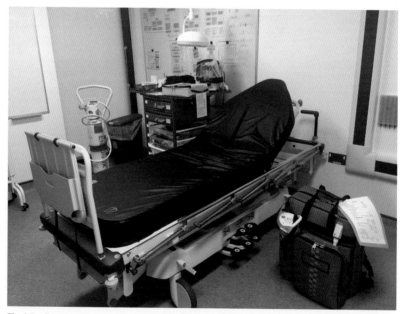

Fig. 2.7 Resuscitation facilities: Advanced life support (ALS) training, equipment and protocols with ALS provision considered in rota planning.

Example Near-patient Investigations

C-reactive protein (CRP):
- Acute-phase reactant; a protein made by the liver and released into the blood within a few hours after tissue injury (example causes include infection, inflammation, myocardial infarction, sepsis, late-stage pregnancy, women taking hormone replacement therapy, obesity)
- *NOT* diagnostic: must be used in conjunction with other factors (signs, symptoms, examination, additional investigations)
- Blood levels less than 10 mg/L are unlikely to be clinically significant
- CRP concentration rises and falls faster than erythrocyte sedimentation rate (ESR)
- Levels rise rapidly within the first 6 to 8 hours and peak after 48 hours

D-Dimer:
- One of the fibrin degradation products from disintegrating clots, normally undetectable
- Significant 'negative predictive value' in excluding venous blood clots, especially in low-risk patients
- No 'positive predictive value' – it is raised in many conditions and does not help to narrow down a differential diagnosis if positive
- Helps exclude, diagnose, and monitor diseases and conditions that cause hypercoagulability, that is, deep vein thrombosis, pulmonary embolism, disseminated intravascular coagulation
- False positives may be associated with recent surgery, trauma, infection, liver or kidney disease, cancers, normal pregnancy and some diseases of pregnancy (i.e. eclampsia), the elderly rheumatoid arthritis, red blood cell rupture (including improper collection and handling)
- False negative value may follow anticoagulation therapy
- Hospital laboratory results are mostly quantitative; near-patient are mostly qualitative

Troponin:
- One of the proteins in muscle fibres that help regulate muscle contraction
- Three different troponins: skeletal muscle troponin C (TnC) and two heart muscle troponins, cardiac troponin T (cTnT) and cardiac troponin I (cTnI)
- Historically: standard cTnI or cTnT test
- Now: high-sensitivity troponins (hs-cTnI or hs-cTnT) detect highly specific markers of heart damage at very low levels
- Biochemical diagnosis of acute heart muscle damage requires an increase in the troponin concentration with time
- Instructions vary according to the specific manufacturer
- If a patient with chest pain and known stable angina has a normal and stable hs-cTn troponin result, it is likely that their heart has not been damaged
- Diagnosis requires a combination of biochemical result, physical examination, clinical history and ECG
- False variable positives (of MI) include: myocarditis, acute heart failure, arrhythmia, chest injury, stroke, PE or pulmonary embolism (blood clot lodged in the lung)
- False constant positives (of MI) include: chronic heart failure, hypertension, kidney disease, severe infections and chronic inflammatory muscle conditions

Personal Protective Equipment and Reducing Healthcare-Associated Infections

NICE has issued guidance aimed at limiting the incidence of healthcare-associated infections (HCAIS)[8] which:
- Arise across a wide range of clinical conditions and can affect patients, healthcare workers, family members and carers

- Can occur in otherwise healthy individuals, especially if invasive procedures or devices are used, that is indwelling urinary catheters
- Are caused by a wide range of microorganisms
- Can exacerbate existing or underlying conditions, delay recovery and adversely affect the quality of life
- Affect 300, 000 patients each year in England as a direct result of care
- Are estimated to cost the NHS approximately £1 billion a year (£56 million of this is estimated to be incurred after patients are discharged from the hospital)

Use of Personal Protective Equipment

Personal protective equipment (PPE) includes a variety of equipment specifically engineered to protect against hazards relating to the clinical workplace and for use in different circumstances, including the use of gloves, aprons, masks, face and eye shields and breathing apparatus. The coronavirus pandemic has highlighted the need for PPE discipline in clinical settings and led to the standard use of PPE such as masks by members of the public to limit disease spread.

When considering PPE use in clinical practice:

- PPE selection, such as that demonstrated in Fig. 2.8, must be based on an assessment of the risk of transmission of microorganisms to the patient, and the risk of contamination of the healthcare worker's clothing and skin by patients' blood, body fluids, secretions or excretions
- Face masks and eye protection must be worn where there is a risk of blood, body fluids, secretions or excretions splashing into the face and eyes
- Respiratory protective equipment, for example, a particulate filter mask, must be used when clinically indicated

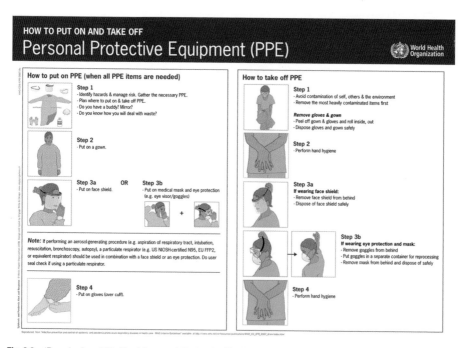

Fig. 2.8 'Donning' and 'Doffing' Personal Protective Equipment (PPE). (From World Health Organization, Geneva, August 2017.)

- Gloves must be worn for invasive procedures, contact with sterile sites and non-intact skin or mucous membranes, and all activities that have been assessed as carrying a risk of exposure to blood, body fluids, secretions or excretions, or to sharp or contaminated instruments
- Gloves must be put on immediately before an episode of patient contact or treatment and removed as soon as the activity is completed
- Gloves must be changed between caring for different patients and between different care or treatment activities for the same patient
- Clinicians should wear:
  - A disposable plastic apron if there is a risk that clothing may be exposed to blood, body fluids, secretions or excretions
  - A long-sleeved fluid-repellent gown if there is a risk of extensive splashing of blood, body fluids, secretions or excretions onto skin or clothing

Indwelling Catheters

Indwelling urinary catheters pose particular concerns regarding HCAIS. Associated principles include:

- Their use should only be considered after alternative methods of management have been considered
- The clinical need for catheterisation should be reviewed regularly and the urinary catheter removed as soon as possible
- Intermittent catheterisation should be used in preference to an indwelling catheter if it is clinically appropriate and a practical option for the patient
- Select the type and gauge of an indwelling urinary catheter based on an assessment of the patient's individual characteristics, including:
  - Age
  - Any allergy or sensitivity to catheter materials
  - Gender (caution – male and female catheters will be of different lengths)
  - History of symptomatic urinary tract infection
  - Patient preference and comfort
  - Previous catheter history
  - Reason for catheterisation
- Typically, the catheter balloon should be inflated with 10 mL of sterile water in adults and 3 to 5 mL in children
- To minimise the risk of blockages, encrustations and catheter-associated infections for patients with a long-term indwelling urinary catheter:
  - Develop a patient-specific care regimen
  - Consider approaches such as reviewing the frequency of planned catheter changes and increasing fluid intake
  - Document catheter blockages
- Antibiotic use when changing indwelling catheters is associated with mixed views regarding antibiotic resistance and patient safety
- When changing catheters in patients with a long-term indwelling urinary catheter:
  - Routine antibiotic prophylaxis is not recommended
  - Consider antibiotic prophylaxis for patients who:
    - Have a history of symptomatic urinary tract infection after catheter change, or
    - Experience trauma during catheterisation

Hand Decontamination

Everyone involved in providing care should be:
- Educated about the standard principles of infection prevention and control
- Trained in hand decontamination, the use of personal protective equipment and the safe use and disposal of sharps
  Wherever care is delivered, healthcare workers must have available appropriate supplies of:
- Materials for hand decontamination
- Sharps containers
- Personal protective equipment
  Hands must be decontaminated:
- Immediately before every episode of direct patient contact or care, including aseptic procedures
- Immediately after every episode of direct patient contact or care
- Immediately after any exposure to body fluids
- Immediately after any other activity or contact with a patient's surroundings that could potentially result in hands becoming contaminated
- Immediately after removal of gloves
  Decontaminate hands preferably with a hand rub except in the following circumstances, when liquid soap and water must be used:
- When hands are visibly soiled or potentially contaminated with body fluids
- In clinical situations where there is potential for the spread of alcohol-resistant organisms (such as *Clostridium difficile* or other organisms that cause diarrheal illness)
  Evidence shows that patients notice when clinical staff fail to wash their hands, yet are not comfortable asking them to do so.[9] Healthcare workers should ensure that their hands can be decontaminated throughout the duration of clinical work by:
- Being bare below the elbow when delivering direct patient care
- Removing wrist and hand jewellery
- Making sure that fingernails are short, clean and free of nail polish
- Covering cuts and abrasions with waterproof dressings

Remote Care and Monitoring

Areas relevant to UUC provision (Fig. 2.9) include:
- Telehealth
  - Video/telephone consultations
  - Desktop, tablets and apps
- Mobile health
  - Medical apps
- Telecare
  - Activity/fall monitoring
  - Remote medication management
- Mobile health
  - Wearables
  - Wellness and fitness apps
  The 'capability' or outcome that can be derived from remote care technology includes:
- Being able to speak 'direct' to patients regardless of location
- Rapid transfer of information, including texting and attachments
- Remote prescribing
- Clinical support to patient contact
- Professional advice/second opinions

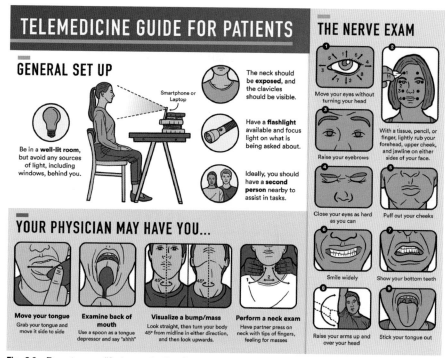

Fig. 2.9 Remote, modified examination in response to the coronavirus pandemic. (Reprinted with permission from Prasad A, Brewster R, Newman JG, et al., 2020.)

- Networked response
- Ongoing follow-up (including using wearable devices)
- The ability to provide a 'networked response', such as that derived using the 'GoodSam' application (Fig. 2.10)[10]

Telemedicine

Advantages to telemedicine include:
- Patient
  - Preference
  - Accessibility
  - Speed
- Clinical
  - Appropriate level of resource
  - Support
  - Second opinions
  - Sub-speciality locations
  - Clinical outcomes
- Operational/Commercial
  - Workforce management/load sharing

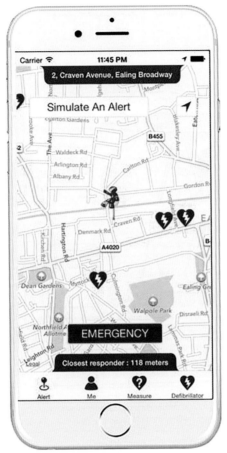

Fig. 2.10 The 'GoodSam' networked response application. (Reproduced with kind permission of GoodSAM.)

- Lone workers
- Remote and rural care
- Cost
- Training and clinical supervision

Challenges to the delivery of telemedicine include:

- General
  - System disruption (to the prevailing NHS clinical footprint of services)
  - Regulation and safety
  - Cost
  - IG and security
  - System inertia (amongst providers, commissioners, practitioners)
- Technical
  - Equipment
  - Technical/situation limitations (weather, signal, etc.)
  - Training and familiarity
  - Availability

- Patients and consultation 'dynamics'
  - Preference
  - Suitability
  - Access/IT literacy
  - Nuances
  - The consultation – communication/examination/investigations
  - Special provisions – safeguarding, capacity etc.
  - Clinical management bias (overuse of antibiotics)
  - Prescribing
- The 'Human Touch'
  - While great advances in terms of networking and shared care may occur, there may also be a reciprocal loss of the special and useful relationships that individual clinicians have with their local patients

Practical considerations when delivering telemedicine:

- Service specification – the commissioner needs to commission it
- Care Quality Commission (CQC) approval – the CQC has issued important advice and guidance for online providers[11]
- Technical – choice of platform/secure video conferencing/appropriate medical records system
- Information governance control
- Use of 'peripherals' to allow remote assessment
- Indemnity
- Equipment governance – the Medicines and Healthcare products Regulatory Agency (MHRA) is the designated competent authority that administers and enforces the law on medical devices in the UK. It has a range of investigatory and enforcement powers to ensure their safety and quality[12]

Clinical safety considerations that the CQC has highlighted include:

- Inappropriate prescribing of antibiotics and prescribing high volumes of opioid-based medicines without reference to the patient's registered general practitioner (GP)
- Unsatisfactory approaches to safeguarding children and those who may not have the mental capacity to understand or consent to a consultation
- Not collecting patient information or sharing information with a patient's NHS GP, or problems that can develop as a result of the fragmentation of medical information
- Inappropriate prescribing of medicines for long-term conditions

References

1. Deloitte. Closing the Digital Gap - Shaping the Future of UK Healthcare. https://www2.deloitte.com/content/dam/Deloitte/uk/Documents/life-sciences-health-care/deloitte-uk-life-sciences-health-care-closing-the-digital-gap.pdf. Accessed 24 May 2020.
2. World Health Organisation. *Health technologies and medicines.* http://www.euro.who.int/en/health-topics/Health-systems/health-technologies-and-medicines. Accessed 24 May 2020.
3. NHSE. *NHS long term plan.* https://www.longtermplan.nhs.uk. Accessed 24 May 2020.
4. NHSE. *NHS digital.* https://digital.nhs.uk. Accessed 24 May 2020.
5. Accenture. *Accenture 2019 digital health consumer survey.* https://www.accenture.com/_acnmedia/PDF-98/Accenture-2019-Digital-Health-Consumer-Survey-ENG.pdf#zoom=50. Accessed 24 May 2020.
6. Hootsuite. *The global state of digital in 2019.* https://hootsuite.com/en-gb/resources/digital-in-2019. Accessed 24 May 2020.
7. NHSE. *Urgent treatment centres – principles and standards.* https://www.england.nhs.uk/publication/urgent-treatment-centres-principles-and-standards/. Accessed 24 May 2020.
8. National Institute for Health and Clinical Excellence. *Infection: prevention and control of healthcare-associated infections in primary and community care.* https://www.nice.org.uk/guidance/cg139/evidence/control-full-guideline-pdf-185186701. Accessed 24 May 2020.

9. McGuckin M, Storr J, Longtin Y, et al. Patient empowerment and multimodal hand hygiene promotion: a win-win strategy. *Am J Med Qual.* 2011;26(1):10–17. https://doi.org/10.1177/1062860610373138.
10. GoodSAM. GoodSAM. https://www.goodsamapp.org. Accessed 24 May 2020.
11. Care Quality Commission. *Clarification of Regulatory Methodology: PMS Digital Healthcare Providers.* https://www.cqc.org.uk/sites/default/files/20170303_pms-digital-healthcare_regulatory-guidance.pdf. Accessed: 24 May 2020.
12. Medicines & Healthcare Products Regulatory Agency. *Medical devices: the regulations and how we enforce them.* https://www.gov.uk/government/publications/report-a-non-compliant-medical-device-enforcement-process/how-mhra-ensures-the-safety-and-quality-of-medical-devices. Accessed 24 May 2020.
13. Hovenga E, Lowe C. *Measuring Capacity To Care Using Nursing Data.* 1st ed. 2020.
14. Prasad A, Brewster R, Newman JG, et al. Optimizing your telemedicine visit during the COVID-19 pandemic: practice guidelines for patients with head and neck cancer. *Head Neck.* 2020;42:1317–1321.

Managing Safe Dispositions

Role and Responsibilities of the Referring Clinician

Referrals are made for a number of reasons, including:

- To establish the diagnosis
- For treatment
- For a specified test or investigation
- For advice on management
- For reassurance
  The King's Fund inquiry into the Quality of General Practice in England[1] noted that:
- Referral often involves a transfer of clinical responsibility between professionals
- It is a complex area where decision-making involves the balancing of several competing concerns and sources of information – not least, the need to respond to patient expectations versus maintaining roles as gatekeepers
- High-quality referral involves the following elements:
  - Necessity – patients are referred as and when necessary, without avoidable delay
  - Destination – patients are referred to the most appropriate place first time
  - Process – the referral process itself is conducted well. For example:
    - Referral letters contain the necessary information, in an accessible format
    - Patients are involved in decision-making around the referral
    - All parties are able to construct a shared understanding of the purpose and expectations of the referral
    - Appropriate investigations and tests are performed prior to referral

- Research evidence indicates that there is scope for quality improvement in referral in terms of each of these dimensions
- Wide variations in referral rates exist, but interpretation of these is highly complex
- Referral rates are influenced by multiple factors – for example, population health needs, attitudes towards risk, and patient pressure
- In order to optimise patient experience and service efficiency, referrals should:
  - Be clinically appropriate for the service referred to
  - Be made in accordance with any agreed clinical pathways and referral protocols
  - Include all the necessary clinical and administrative information

De-escalating Situations

Context of increasing concerns regarding the safety of clinicians, staff and other patients by violent or threatening patients. Factors that influence and trigger violence in patients may include:
- Fear
- Pain
- Frustration
- Threat (real or perceived)
- Criminal behaviour (not explained by situation or clinical state)
- Prevailing factors (stress, anxiety, general situation)
- Cultural factors including language difficulties, differences in values and beliefs
- Combination of verbal and nonverbal cues
  Patient behaviour and presentation that may indicate anger and imminent violence include:
- Angry and irritable behaviour
- Hyperactivity including restlessness, twitching, pacing, gesticulating
- Patterns of tension and anxiety including clenched jaw and fist, tense facial expression, flushing, sweating, tremor
- Shouting or raised voice, verbal abuse, swearing, threatening
- Change of pitch or soft voice
- Avoidance of eye contact or intense eye contact and staring
- Invading of personal space
- Withdrawal and silence
- Alcohol or drug intoxication
- Disordered thoughts, suspicious thinking and rumination
  Environments that may exacerbate the situation include:
- Hot, noisy, crowded areas
- Harsh lighting
- Poor access and long waits
- Poor signage and layout
- Badly controlled/poorly staffed areas where there seems to be little control and staff have not been taught de-escalation techniques
- Lack of policies and equipment (panic buttons, etc.)
- Presence of security team (generally a good thing)
- Facilities where bad behaviour has been previously tolerated and not challenged (including that of other patients)
  Considerations include:
- Always consider safety and personal competence to deal with the situation
- Summon immediate help when needed
- Avoid confrontation and stand-offs
- Consider both verbal and nonverbal and cues
- Re-assess patient's response to de-escalation techniques

Measures to de-escalate include:

General

- Face the person/facing away at slight angle
- Calm demeanour
- Reasonable eye contact
- Smiling and reassuring
- Active listening
- Slow pace
- Protect personal space
- Smile
- Avoid provocation

Verbal

- Introduce yourself
- Calm, gentle tone
- Use patient's name frequently
- Active listening with minimal interruptions
- Identify and acknowledge feelings, concerns and wants
- Simplify where possible
- Remain positive and supportive
- Try to seek common ground
- Distract where necessary
- Use understanding phrases, that is 'that must have been difficult', 'we'd like to do what we can to help you'
- Offer to help but explain (imposed) boundaries

Factors Influencing Referral Decisions

The same King's Fund inquiry identified that the following factors influenced referral decisions:

- Individuals' variation between different clinicians in terms of their diagnostic and referral practices
- The complexity of diagnosis and referral and factors influencing them
- Clinical relationships which facilitate information exchange, provide learning opportunities and underpin high-quality diagnosis and referral.
- The GP–patient relationship and the quality of the consultation
  The inquiry made the following related recommendations:
- A naïve pursuit of standardisation could be dangerous, and should not be encouraged
- There is scope for quality measurement in diagnosis and referral, but most indicators (such as referral rates) should be used to prompt further investigation rather than as an unambiguous marker of performance
- Mechanisms and incentives for improving communication between those making and receiving referrals should be explored
- Good relationships may also make it easier to seek informal advice, reducing the need for making formal referrals and avoiding duplication of tests
- A stronger clinical governance framework is needed to better understand and improve the quality of clinical decision-making
- Longer consultation times could be expected to support improved decision-making around diagnosis and referral
- More research is needed to link diagnostic and referral practices with clinical outcomes

Factors Influencing Risk-based Decision-making

Clinicians weigh up numerous factors in reaching conclusions such as those captured in Fig. 3.1. The nature of their decision-making centres around[2]:

- 'What is the problem?'
- 'What are the possible solutions?'
- 'What is the best solution for this patient?'

Numerous models are used to describe the diagnostic process, one of this (the 'hypotheticodeductive model') breaks it down into the following steps:

- Information gathering
- Hypothesis generation
- Hypothesis testing
- Reflection

A BMJ study looking at GPs working in out-of-hours primary care found that the most powerful themes in terms of decision making related to[3]:

- Dealing with urgent potentially high-risk cases
- Keeping patients safe and responding to their needs
- While trying to keep patients out of hospital and the concept of 'fire-fighting'

Specific characteristics made decision-making more easy or difficult to deal with:

- Severely ill patients were straightforward
- Older people with complex multi-system diseases were often difficult

GPs stopped collecting clinical information and came to clinical decisions when:

- High-risk disease and severe illness requiring hospital attention has been excluded
- They had responded directly to the patient's needs
- There was a reliable safety net in place

Learning points that GPs identified as important for trainees in the out-of-hours setting included:

- The importance of developing rapport despite time pressures
- Learning to deal with uncertainty
- Learning about common presentations with a focus on critical cues to exclude severe illness

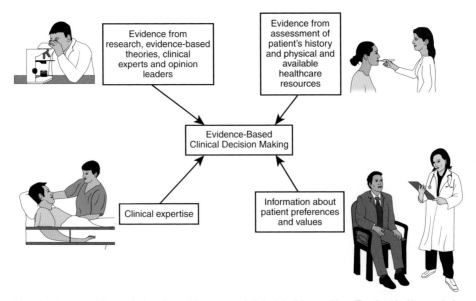

Fig. 3.1 Example of factors influencing evidence-based clinical decision-making. (Reprinted with permission from Potter PA et al., 2017.)

Decision-making and Referral in Remote Consultation

Remote consultations confer particular challenges and clinical risks, which include:

- Disrupted ('unnatural') conversation
- Loss of nuances and nonverbal cues
- Reduced clinical examination/assessment including physiological observations
- Impaired consultation flow – communication/examination/investigation
- Clinical management bias (i.e. overuse of antibiotics to ensure important diagnoses are not missed)
- Potential for patient manipulation – i.e. drug-seeking behaviour
- More limited ability to pick up important information – i.e. safeguarding, capacity
- Prescribing bias i.e. antibiotic thresholds

Clinical safety considerations that the Care Quality Commission (CQC) has highlighted include:

- Inappropriate prescribing of antibiotics and prescribing high volumes of opioid-based medicines without reference to the patient's registered GP
- Unsatisfactory approaches to safeguarding children and those who may not have the mental capacity to understand or consent to a consultation
- Not collecting patient information or sharing information with a patient's NHS GP, or problems that can develop as a result of the fragmentation of medical information
- Inappropriate prescribing of medicines for long-term conditions

Remote Consultations – Safeguarding Considerations

The delivery of remote/video medical care poses several particular safeguarding considerations that include but are not limited to:

- The potential that 'opportunistic' or subtle safeguarding presentations, signs and symptoms may be missed
- Patients may be less willing to volunteer important and difficult information through this format
- Remote clinicians may be less familiar with safeguarding procedure variations across multiple sites
- Remote clinicians may assume that local safeguarding systems will be in place or activated
- A time delay may be introduced between termination of the consultation and communication of outcome to the registered general practitioner
- Some patients may use the service but not be registered with a GP
- The potential for individuals (or 'controlling parties') to use the remote format as a way of accessing medical care without alerting medical suspicion of abuse
- The potential for individuals (or 'controlling parties') to use the remote format as a way of trying to gain access to inappropriate care or potential medicines of abuse
- The management of a remote and geographically diverse workforce
- Less continuity of care

Supportive Care and Avoiding Admissions

Twenty percent to 25% of admissions and 50% of bed days do not require an 'acute' hospital bed, while 39% of people delayed in hospital could have been discharged using different pathways. Unnecessarily prolonged stays in hospital are bad for patients and the system, because[4]:

- They cause unnecessary waiting, sleep deprivation, increased risk of falls and fracture, prolonging episodes of acute confusion (delirium) and catching healthcare-associated infections

- They can cause an avoidable loss of muscle strength leading to greater physical dependency (commonly referred to as de-conditioning); 35% of 70-year-old patients experience functional decline during hospital admission in comparison with their pre-illness baseline; for people over 90 this increases to 65%
- Are costly
- Can cause hospital-related functional decline in older patients
- A stay in hospital over 10 days leads to 10 years of muscle ageing for some people who are most at risk

Congested hospitals struggle to deliver best care; reducing bed occupancy to improve flow through the system greatly improves the working and care environment, reduces A&E crowding and enables patients consistently to be treated in the right bed by clinical teams with the right skills. The emergency Care Improvement Programme directs that '6 As' should be used to avoid admissions[5]:

- Advice – suggest a clinical management plan that allows the patient to be managed in primary care
- Access outpatient services – suggest an outpatient referral for specialist assessment
- Ambulatory Emergency Care – clinically stable patients appropriate for same-day discharge
- Acute Frailty Unit – to provide comprehensive geriatric assessment for frail older patients
- Acute Assessment Units – to diagnose and stabilise patients likely to need admission
- Admission to speciality ward directly – for agreed clinical pathways and specialised clinical presentations

Ambulatory Emergency Units are important elements of the UUC pathway that have the following characteristics:

- Offer same-day emergency care for patients being considered for emergency admission
- Reduce inpatient admissions by providing early senior assessment and intervention
- Are safe, well-accepted by patients and highly cost-effective
- Have considerable impact; a properly resourced and implemented service can reduce inpatient admissions by up to 30%
- Must not be used during escalation for inpatient admissions as doing so will exacerbate hospital crowding rather than reduce it
- Works best with effective streaming in the emergency department
- Best practice involves a clinical discussion between an emergency department clinical decision-maker or the patient's GP and the ambulatory emergency care (AEC) team ahead of referral

The King's Fund looked at evidence actually regarding admissions avoidance, finding[6]:

- Conditions that are most avoidable are ambulatory or primary care-sensitive conditions
- Some admissions (e.g. those for dementia) may not be perceived to be avoidable, as the disease course is not significantly modifiable, but the availability of more suitable alternatives to an acute hospital admission (e.g. respite care or home care) can result in admission avoidance in the acute situation
- Interventions where there is evidence of positive effect on reducing admissions include:
  - Continuity of care with a GP
  - Hospital at home as an alternative to admission
  - Assertive case management in mental health
  - Self-management
  - Early senior review in A&E
  - Multidisciplinary interventions
  - Tele-monitoring in heart failure
  - Integration of primary and secondary care

- Interventions with evidence of little or no beneficial effect include:
  - Pharmacist home-based medication review
  - Intermediate care
  - Community-based case management (generic conditions)
  - Early discharge to hospital at home on readmissions
  - Nurse-led interventions pre- and post-discharge for patients with chronic obstructive pulmonary disease (COPD)
- Interventions for which further evidence is needed include:
  - Increasing GP practice size
  - Changing out-of-hours primary care arrangements
  - Chronic care management in primary care
  - Telemedicine
  - Cost-effectiveness of GPs in A&E
  - Access to social care in A&E
  - Hospital-based case management
  - Rehabilitation programmes
  - Rapid response teams

Compulsory Mental Health Admission in England

Admission
- Great majority of patients admitted to mental health hospitals are admitted informally
- Compulsory detention would occur if a person is so unwell that it is considered to be in the interest of their health or safety, or for the protection of others for a period of time, for assessment or treatment.

Procedure
- When two doctors and an Approved Mental Health Professional (AMHP) have all agreed that admission is appropriate and necessary
- At least one of the doctors must be approved under the Mental Health Act (most likely to be a psychiatrist) and, if possible, at least one of the doctors should already have previous knowledge of the person
- In order to provide sufficient authority for a compulsory admission, both doctors must make a medical recommendation and the AMHP must make an application
- This also provides the authority to convey the person to hospital, where they can be detained for a specific period
- If both doctors recommend detention in hospital, but the AMHP is unwilling to make an application, the person's nearest relative may make the application, and the AMHP will be required to facilitate the admission to hospital

Admission for Assessment – Section 2
- Can be detained under Section 2 of the Mental Health Act for up to 28 days, but not necessarily for the whole of the 28-day period
- At the end of this period, if further detention is considered necessary, an assessment for Section 3 would need to be carried out

Admission for Treatment – Section 3
- Can be detailed under this section for up to 6 months, but not necessarily for the whole of this period
- At the end of this period, if the person is considered to need further treatment, the detention can be renewed for a further 6-month period, and thereafter for periods of 12 months

Community Treatment Order (CTO)
- Can be used for people who have been detained in hospital for treatment, where the responsible clinician (RC) considers that the person requires further treatment, which

doesn't need to take place in a hospital setting, but the person is unlikely to comply with their treatment in the community in the absence of a CTO
- Come with conditions to promote the person's ongoing treatment and recovery
- Failure to comply with these conditions can result in being recalled to hospitals where the original detention for treatment can be reinstated.

Emergency Admission – Section 4
- In an emergency situation, a person can be detained for up to 72 hours based on only one medical recommendation and an application, during which time another doctor may complete the second recommendation necessary for a Section 2

Discharge
- The RC in overall charge of the patient's assessment or treatment may discharge the patient from detention at any time
- The nearest relative may also discharge the patient from detention by giving 72 hours' notice in writing to the hospital managers
- During the notice period, the RC may overrule the nearest relative, in which case detention continues to apply
- Once discharged from detention, if the RC agrees, the person may remain in the hospital as an informal patient for further assessment or treatment.

The Mental Capacity Act (MCA) 2005

Five principles underpin the MCA. In order to protect those who lack capacity and to enable them to take part, as much as possible in decisions that affect them, the following statutory principles apply:
- You must always assume a person has capacity unless it is proved otherwise
- You must take all practicable steps to enable people to make their own decisions
- You must not assume incapacity simply because someone makes an unwise decision
- Always act, or decide, for a person without capacity in their best interests
- Carefully consider actions to ensure the least restrictive option is taken

Assessment of Capacity

Follow the 2-stage test for capacity (failure on one point will determine lack of capacity)[7]:
- Stage 1: Does the person have an impairment of the mind or brain (temporary or permanent)?
- Stage 2: Is the person able to:
  - Understand the decision they need to make and why they need to make it?
  - Understand, retain, use and weigh information relevant to the decision?
  - Understand the consequences of making, or not making, this decision?
  - Communicate their decision by any means (i.e. speech, sign language)?
  In order to act in someone's best interests you should:
- Avoid making assumptions about capacity based on age, appearance or medical condition
- Encourage the person to participate as fully as possible
- Consider whether the person will in the future have capacity in relation to the matter in question
- Consider the person's past and present beliefs, values, wishes and feelings
- Take into account the views of others – that is carers, relatives, friends, advocates
- Consider the least restrictive options
- Use Best Interests checklists as part of local policy and procedure and the MCA Code of Practice

In addition, you should also consider:

- The MCA Code of Practice: Professionals and carers must have regard to the Code and record reasons for assessing capacity or best interests. If anyone decides to depart from the Code they must record their reasons for doing so
- LPAs & ADs: Is there a valid/current Lasting Power of Attorney (LPA) or an Advance Decision (AD) in place?
- IMCAs: The MCA set up a service, the Independent Mental Capacity Advocate (IMCA), to help vulnerable people who lack capacity and are facing important decisions including serious healthcare treatment decisions and who have no one else to speak for them
- Are the decisions being taken in the person's best interests, the least restrictive option? Consider whether an authorisation is required to deprive the person of their liberty?

In emergency situations, where there may not always be time for all investigation and consultation:

- There should be no liability for acting in the reasonable belief that someone lacks capacity, and what you do is reasonably believed to be in their best interests
- This can include restraint if need be, if it is proportionate and necessary to prevent harm to the patient, and even 'a deprivation of liberty', if this is necessary for 'life sustaining treatment or a vital act', while a Court Order is sought if needed

Deprivation of Liberty Safeguards

General principles:

- Deprivation of Liberty Safeguards 2009 (DoLS) is an amendment to the Mental Capacity Act 2005
- They provide a legal framework to protect those who lack the capacity to consent to the arrangements for their treatment or care (e.g. by reason of their dementia, learning disability or brain injury) and where levels of restriction or restraint used in delivering that care for the purpose of protection from risk/harm are so extensive as to potentially be depriving the person of their liberty
- Sometimes a deprivation of liberty (DoL) is required to provide care/treatment and protect people from harm, but every effort should be made to ensure care is delivered in the least restrictive environment possible
- If a DoL cannot be avoided, it should be for no longer than is necessary
- CCGs and Local Authorities are required to apply to the Court of Protection to have the application for DoL authorised
- DoLs can relate to individuals in hospitals, care homes, residential and nursing homes (i.e. all CQC registered settings) – currently, the provider organisation is required to apply to the Local Authority where the patient is from, to have the application for DoL authorised

An application is required to the Court of Protection where the following conditions are met:

- The person has an impairment or disturbance in the functioning of their mind or brain which could affect their ability to make a decision
- The person does not have the capacity to consent to their circumstances/care arrangements and/or treatment
- Their situation meets the acid test that they are 'under continuous supervision and control and are not free to leave'

Child Safeguarding

Overarching Acts and Standards include:

- The Care Act 2014
- CQC's Essential Standards of Quality and Safety
- NHS England's 'Safeguarding vulnerable people in the reformed NHS; accountability and assurance framework 2015'
- United Nations Convention on the Rights of the Child
- Children Act 1989
- Equality Act 2010
  Two key principles underpin all effective safeguarding arrangements for children:
- Safeguarding is everyone's responsibility; for services to be effective, each professional organisation should play their full part
- A child-centred approach: for services to be effective they need to be based on a clear understanding of the needs and views of children.
  Safeguarding and promoting the welfare of children means:
- Protecting children from maltreatment
- Preventing impairment of children's health and development
- Ensuring that children grow up in circumstances consistent with the provision of safe and effective care
- Taking action to enable all children to have the best outcomes
  Types of abuse and neglect relating more to children[8]:
- Abuse – a form of maltreatment of a child. Somebody may abuse or neglect a child by inflicting harm or by failing to act to prevent harm. Children may be abused in a family or in an institutional or community setting by those known to them or, more rarely, by others (e.g. via the Internet). They may be abused by an adult or adults, or another child or children
- Physical abuse – a form of abuse which may involve hitting, shaking, throwing, poisoning, burning or scalding, drowning, suffocating or otherwise causing physical harm to a child. Physical harm may also be caused when a parent or carer fabricates the symptoms of, or deliberately induces, illness in a child
- Emotional abuse – the persistent emotional maltreatment of a child such as to cause severe and persistent adverse effects on the child's emotional development. It may involve conveying to a child that they are worthless or unloved, inadequate, or valued only insofar as they meet the needs of another person. It may include not giving the child opportunities to express their views, deliberately silencing them or 'making fun' of what they say or how they communicate. It may feature age or developmentally inappropriate expectations being imposed on children. These may include interactions that are beyond a child's developmental capability as well as overprotection and limitation of exploration and learning, or preventing the child participating in normal social interaction. It may involve seeing or hearing the ill-treatment of another. It may involve serious bullying (including cyber bullying), causing children frequently to feel frightened or in danger, or the exploitation or corruption of children. Some level of emotional abuse is involved in all types of maltreatment of a child, though it may occur alone
- Sexual abuse – involves forcing or enticing a child or young person to take part in sexual activities, not necessarily involving a high level of violence, whether or not the child is aware of what is happening. The activities may involve physical contact, including assault by penetration (e.g. rape or oral sex) or non-penetrative acts such as masturbation, kissing, rubbing and touching outside of clothing. They may also include non-contact activities, such as involving children in looking at, or in the production of, sexual images, watching sexual activities, encouraging children to behave in sexually inappropriate ways, or grooming a child

in preparation for abuse (including via the Internet). Sexual abuse is not solely perpetrated by adult males. Women can also commit acts of sexual abuse, as can other children
- Neglect – the persistent failure to meet a child's basic physical and/or psychological needs, likely to result in the serious impairment of the child's health or development. Neglect may occur during pregnancy as a result of maternal substance abuse. Once a child is born, neglect may involve a parent or carer failing to: provide adequate food, clothing and shelter (including exclusion from home or abandonment); protect a child from physical and emotional harm or danger; ensure adequate supervision (including the use of inadequate care-givers); or ensure access to appropriate medical care or treatment.

Adult Safeguarding

An adult at risk is defined as any person aged 18 years and over who[9]:
- Has needs for care or support (whether or not the Local Authority is meeting those needs);
- Is experiencing, or is at risk of, abuse and neglect; and
- As a result of those care and support needs is unable to protect themselves from either, the risk of, or the experience of, abuse or neglect.

Six principles underpin all safeguarding work for adults.[10] These principles apply across all sectors and settings:
- Empowerment – people being supported and encouraged to make their own decisions and informed consent
- Prevention – it is better to take action before harm occurs
- Proportionality – the least intrusive response appropriate to the risk presented
- Protection – support and representation for those in greatest need
- Partnership – local solutions through services working with their communities. Communities have a part to play in preventing, detecting and reporting abuse and neglect
- Accountability – accountability and transparency in delivering safeguarding
  Types of abuse and neglect relating more to adults:
- Physical abuse – including assault, hitting, slapping, pushing, misuse of medication, restraint or inappropriate physical sanctions
- Domestic violence – including psychological, physical, sexual, financial, emotional abuse; so called 'honour' based violence
- Sexual abuse – including rape, indecent exposure, sexual harassment, inappropriate looking or touching, sexual teasing or innuendo, sexual photography, subjection to pornography or witnessing sexual acts, indecent exposure and sexual assault or sexual acts to which the adult has not consented or was pressured into consenting
- Psychological abuse – including emotional abuse, threats of harm or abandonment, deprivation of contact, humiliation, blaming, controlling, intimidation, coercion, harassment, verbal abuse, cyber bullying, isolation or unreasonable and unjustified withdrawal of services or supportive networks
- Financial or material abuse – including theft, fraud, Internet scamming, coercion in relation to an adult's financial affairs or arrangements, including in connection with wills, property, inheritance or financial transactions, or the misuse or misappropriation of property, possessions or benefits
- Modern slavery – encompasses slavery, human trafficking, forced labour and domestic servitude. Traffickers and slave masters use whatever means they have at their disposal to coerce, deceive and force individuals into a life of abuse, servitude and inhumane treatment.
  - Discriminatory abuse – including forms of harassment, slurs or similar treatment; because of race, gender and gender identity, age, disability, sexual orientation or religion

- Organisational abuse – including neglect and poor care practice within an institution or specific care setting such as a hospital or care home, for example, in relation to care provided in one's own home. This may range from one off incidents to ongoing ill-treatment. It can be through neglect or poor professional practice as a result of the structure, policies, processes and practices within an organisation
- Neglect and acts of omission – including ignoring medical, emotional or physical care needs, failure to provide access to appropriate health, care and support or educational services, the withholding of the necessities of life, such as medication, adequate nutrition and heating
- Self-neglect – this covers a wide range of behaviour neglecting to care for one's personal hygiene, health or surroundings and includes behaviour such as hoarding

Assessment should occur using a thorough, holistic assessment which considers wider points of information including:

- The patient's views and wishes
- Inconsistencies in the history or explanation
- Personal presentation such as being unkempt
- Delays or evidence of obstacles in seeking or receiving treatment
- Evidence of frequent attendances to health services including seeking remote care
- Consideration of capacity for the decision required
- The ability to give informed consent
- Others potentially at-risk individuals, for example children or other vulnerable adults
- Whether immediate protection required
- Whether a crime has been committed and the police should be informed
- Whether other agencies are involved

Raising Concerns

Where abuse is suspected the safety and welfare of the patient or person involved is the first priority. The immediate situation should be made safe and efforts made to ensure that support will be provided for the individual. If it is clear that a crime has been committed, then the police must be informed.

The pneumonic **CRASH** (Fig. 3.2) is a useful framework:

- **C**onsider: the chance there could be a safeguarding issue
- **R**ecognise: be alert for vulnerable patients
- **A**ct: follow your protocols and inform necessary parties
- **S**ecure: confirm reports have been submitted and received
- **H**ousekeeping: follow up, debrief, audit

Consider the following principles regarding information sharing:

- Where there are safeguarding concerns, staff have a *duty* to share information
- In most serious case reviews, lack of information sharing can be a significant contributor when things go wrong
- Information should be shared with consent wherever possible
- A person's right to confidentiality is not absolute and may be overridden where there is evidence that sharing information is necessary to support an investigation or where there is a risk to others, for example in the interests of public safety, police investigation, implications for regulated service
- The Data Protection Act (DPA) is not a barrier to sharing information but provides a framework to ensure that personal information about living persons is shared appropriately
- Be open and honest with the person (and/or their family where appropriate) from the outset about why, what, how and with whom information will or could be shared and seek their agreement, unless it is unsafe or inappropriate to do so

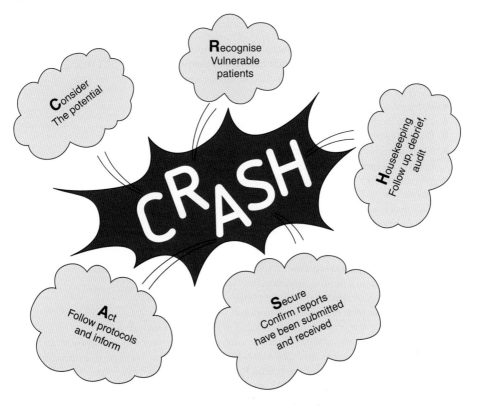

Fig. 3.2 'CRASH' safeguarding considerations.

- Seek advice if you are in any doubt, without disclosing the identity of the person where possible
- Share with consent where appropriate and, where possible, respect the wishes of those who do not consent to share confidential information. You may still share information without consent if, in your judgement, that lack of consent can be overridden in the public interest. You will need to base your judgement on the facts of the case
- Consider safety and well-being: base your information sharing decisions on considerations of the safety and well-being of the person and others who may be affected by their actions or the actions of the perpetrator
- Sharing should be necessary, proportionate, relevant, accurate, timely and secure: Ensure that the information you share is necessary for the purpose for which you are sharing it, is shared only with those people who need to have it, is accurate and up-to-date, is shared in a timely fashion and is shared securely
- Keep a record of your decision and the reasons for it – whether it is to share information or not. If you decide to share, then record what you have shared, with whom and for what purpose

Whistle Blowing

- *Always act* whenever abuse is suspected including when your legitimate concern is not acted upon
- Whistle blowers are given protection under the Public Interest Disclosure Act 1998

Prevent/Channel

Prevent is the part of the government's counter-terrorism strategy (known as CONTEST) which aims to stop people becoming terrorists or supporting terrorism.[11] The strategy promotes collaboration and co-operation among public service organisations.

CONTEST has four key principles:

- Pursue: to stop terrorist attacks
- Prevent: to stop people becoming terrorists or supporting terrorism
- Protect: to strengthen our protection against a terrorist attack
- Prepare: to mitigate the impact of a terrorist attack

Healthcare workers have a key part to play since:

- Prevent focuses on working with vulnerable individuals who may be at risk of being exploited by radicalisers and subsequently drawn into terrorist-related activity
- They may identify people and behaviour before it becomes criminal
- Collaborative working adds real value to patient care

Practical steps include:

- Noticing unusual changes in the behaviour of patients and/or colleagues
- Knowing how to raise concerns
- Attending prevent training and awareness programmes
- Being aware of professional responsibilities
- Being familiar with organisational protocols

Factors that might make people vulnerable to exploitation include:

- Identity crisis – adolescents/vulnerable adults exploring issues of identity can feel both distant from their parents/family and cultural and religious heritage and uncomfortable with their place in society around them. Radicalisers can exploit this by providing a sense of purpose or feelings of belonging. Where this occurs, it can often manifest itself in a change in a person's behaviour, their circle of friends, and the way in which they interact with others and spend their time
- Personal crisis – may include significant tensions within the family that produce a sense of isolation of the vulnerable individual from the traditional certainties of family life
- Personal circumstances – individuals may perceive their aspirations for career and lifestyle to be undermined by limited achievements or employment prospects. This can translate to a generalised rejection of civic life and adoption of violence as a symbolic act
- Criminality – in some cases, a vulnerable individual may have been involved in a group that engages in criminal activity or, on occasion, a group that has links to organised crime and be further drawn to engagement in terrorist-related activity
- Grievances – which may play an important part in the early indoctrination of vulnerable individuals into the acceptance of a radical view and extremist ideology
- A misconception and/or rejection of UK foreign policy
- Distrust of western media reporting
- Perceptions that UK government policy is discriminatory (e.g. counter-terrorist legislation)
- Other factors such as:
  - Ideology and politics
  - Provocation and anger (grievance)
  - Need for protection
  - Seeking excitement and action
  - Fascination with violence, weapons and uniforms
  - Youth rebellion
  - Seeking family and father substitutes
  - Seeking friends and community
  - Seeking status and identity

- Other signs:
  - Parental/family reports of unusual changes in behaviour, friendships or actions and requests for assistance
  - Patients/staff accessing extremist material online
  - Use of extremist or hate terms to exclude others or incite violence
  - Writing or artwork promoting violent extremist messages or images

Domestic Violence and Abuse

Domestic violence and abuse are officially classified as 'any incident of threatening behaviours, violence or abuse between adults who are or have been in a relationship together, or between family members, regardless of gender or sexuality'. The statistics are alarming:
- One woman in three (and one man in five) in the United Kingdom will be a victim of domestic violence during their lifetime
- Two women a week are killed by a current or former male partner.
  Key principles for those encountering service users that may have been victims of domestic violence or sexual abuse:
- Act – never assume someone else is addressing the domestic violence and abuse issues
- Respect – remember it is not the professional's role to comment on or encourage a person experiencing abuse to leave their partner
- Revisit – if a patient does not disclose but you suspect otherwise, accept what is being said but offer other opportunities to talk and consider giving information (e.g. 'for a friend')
- Act – share information appropriately subject to policy and local guidance
  When asking about domestic abuse[12]:
- Ensure it is safe to ask
- Consider the environment:
  - Is it conducive to ask?
  - Is it safe to ask?
  - Never ask in the presence of another family member, friend or child over the age of 2 years (or any other persons including a partner)
- Create the opportunity to ask the question
- Use an appropriate professional interpreter (never a family member)
- Frame the topic first then ask a direct question
- Validate what's happening to the individual and send important messages to the contact:
  - 'You are not alone'
  - 'You are not to blame for what is happening to you'
  - 'You do not deserve to be treated in this way'
- Assess contact safety:
  - 'Is your partner here with you?'
  - 'Where are the children?'
  - 'Do you have any immediate concerns?'
  - 'Do you have a place of safety?'
- Consider safety and confidentiality when recording information in patient notes (not in patient-held record)
- Medical records can be used by survivors in future criminal justice proceedings.

Human Trafficking

Human Trafficking involves men, women and children being brought into a situation of exploitation through the use of violence, deception or coercion and forced to work against their will.[13] People can be trafficked for many different forms of exploitation such as forced prostitution, forced labour, forced begging, and forced criminality, domestic servitude, forced marriage, forced organ removal. When children are trafficked, no violence, deception or coercion needs to be involved: simply bringing them into exploitative conditions constitutes trafficking.

People trafficking and people smuggling are often confused:

- People smuggling is the illegal movement of people across international border for a fee and upon arrival in the country of destination the smuggled person is free
- The trafficking of people is fundamentally different as the trafficker is facilitating the movement of that person for the purpose of exploitation
- There is no need for an international border to be crossed in cases of trafficking, it occurs also nationally, even within one community

If you suspect human trafficking/modern slavery, contact '101' to report your information

Modern Slavery

Modern slavery is:

- The illegal exploitation of people for personal/ commercial gain
- Victims trapped in servitude they were deceived or coerced into
- Criminal exploitation: pick pocketing, shop-lifting, drug trafficking
- Domestic servitude: forced to work in private houses with restricted freedoms, long hours, no pay
- Forced labour: long hours, no pay, poor conditions, verbal and physical threats
- Sexual exploitation: prostitution and child abuse
- Other forms: organ removal, forced begging, forced marriage and illegal adoption
  Signs of modern slavery may include:
- Look malnourished or unkempt
- Withdrawn, anxious and unwilling to interact
- Under the control and influence of others
- Live in cramped, dirty, overcrowded accommodation
- No access or control of their passport or identity documents, or use false or forged documents
- Appear scared, avoid eye contact and be untrusting
- Show signs of abuse and/or have health issues
- Show old/untreated injuries, or delay seeking medical care with vague/inconsistent explanation for injuries
- Appear to wear the same or unsuitable clothes, with few personal possessions
- Fear authorities and in fear of removal or consequences for family
- In debt to others or a situation of dependence

Female Genital Mutilation

Female genital mutilation (FGM) is child abuse. It:

- Causes significant harm and constitutes physical and emotional abuse
- Is a violation of a child's bodily integrity as well as their right to health
- Is against the law in the United Kingdom and has been a criminal offence since 1985
- Is a serious crime that carries a penalty of 14 years in prison
- It is an offence to make arrangements for FGM to be undertaken within the United Kingdom or to take, or plan to take a child out of the United Kingdom for the purpose of FGM
  If you are concerned that FGM has or may happen:
- It is a mandatory duty for a regulated healthcare professional to report concerns about a female under 18 years and record when FGM is disclosed or identified as part of NHS healthcare

- The duty is a personal duty which requires the individual professional who becomes aware of the case to make a report; the responsibility cannot be transferred
- As FGM is illegal this should be reported to the Police
  Female genital mutilation[14]:
- Comprises all procedures involving partial or total removal of the external female genital organs or any other injury to the female genital organs for non-medical reasons
- Is most often carried out on young girls aged between infancy and 15 years old
- Is often referred to as 'cutting', 'female circumcision', 'initiation', 'Sunna' and 'infibulation'.
  FGM in the United Kingdom:
- An estimated 65,000 girls aged 13 and under are at risk of FGM in the United Kingdom
- UK communities most at risk include Kenyan, Somalian, Sudanese, Sierra Leonean, Egyptian, Nigerian and Eritrean
- Non-African countries that practise FGM include Yemen, Afghanistan, Kurdistan, Indonesia, Malaysia, Turkey, Thailand (South) and Pakistani
- There is a need to consider whether it has or may occur
  Signs that should alert suspicions regarding FGM risk include:
- Knowing that a mother or older sibling has undergone FGM
- A girl talking about plans to have a 'special procedure' or to attend a special occasion/ celebration to 'become a woman'
- A girl's parents saying that they or a relative will take the child out of the country for a prolonged period, or school holidays or when attending for travel vaccinations
- A girl may talk about a long holiday to her country of origin or another country where the practice is present
- The girl is a member of the community that is less integrated into UK society and whose country of origin practices FGM.
  Signs that a child may have already undergone FGM:
- Difficultly walking, sitting or standing
- Spending longer than normal in the bathroom or toilet due to difficulties urinating
- Soreness, infection or unusual presentation noticed by practitioner when changing a nappy or helping with toileting
- Spending long periods of time away from the classroom during the day with bladder or menstrual problems
- Having frequent unusual menstrual problems
- Prolonged or repeated absence from school or college
- A prolonged absence from school or college with personal or behaviour changes, for example withdrawn, depressed
- Being particularly reluctant to undergo normal medical examinations
- Asking for help or advice but not being explicit about the procedure due to embarrassment or fear

Patient Transfer and Transport

The intercollegiate board for pre-hospital emergency medicine (PHEM) curriculum describes 'transfer' as 'the process of transporting a patient while maintaining in-transit clinical care'[15]:

- A distinction between retrieval and transport (or transfer) is sometimes made on the basis of the location of the patient (e.g. scene or hospital) and the composition or origins of the retrieval or transfer team
- Successful pre-hospital emergency medical services recognise that many of the competencies required to primarily transport critically ill or injured patients from the incident scene to hospital are the same as those required for secondary intra-hospital or inter-hospital transport

Potential reasons to transfer a patient include:
- Transfer for specialist care and investigation
- Transfer for non-clinical reasons (lack of resources, lack of critical care beds, inadequate staffing levels)
- Repatriation – to move a patient for care closer to home

Modes of transport are determined by:
- Urgency of the transfer
- Condition of the patient
- Geographical factors
- Weather conditions
- Traffic
- Availability
- Suitable landing sites at destination, including secondary landing site to hospital and availability of vehicle (where required)
- Distance

Pre-transfer actions should/could include:
- Familiarisation with treatment already undertaken
- Independently assess the patient's condition
- Risk assessment
- Appropriate resuscitation and stabilisation prior to transfer
- Re-checking of all equipment and drugs
- Cannulate placement
- Chest drain placement
- Nasogastric tubes
- Urinary catheters
- Departure check lists

In-transfer monitoring may include:
- Basic observations
- Pain scores
- ECG-continuous
- Non-invasive blood pressure
- Pulse oximetry (SpO_2)
- End-tidal carbon dioxide ($EtCO_2$) in ventilated patients
- Temperature
- Airway pressure monitor in ventilated patients

In-transfer management should include:
- Keeping patient warm
- Protect eyes, ears and pressure areas
- Secure using transfer trolley by means of a 5-point harness or similar
- Monitor patient continuously throughout the transfer
- Keep monitors, ventilator and pumps visible at all times
- Normally high-speed travel is not necessary
- The decision to use blue lights and/or police escort rests with the ambulance crew who will take advice from the senior clinician on board
- Remaining seated at all times and wear seat belts

Formal handovers (inter-hospital scenario):
- Must occur between the transfer team and the receiving nurses and medical staff
- Must include written records
- Should include: presentation and course; past medical history; results of investigations; list of current medications and doses; contact details of referring team
- Should take place in a calm environment once the patient is settled

Role of Clinicians in Transfers

Areas that clinicians need to consider for transfers include[16]:
- Transfer decisions and ethics
- Communication with patients and relatives
- Selection of transport mode
- Accompanying personnel and risk assessment
- Preparation for transport
- Use of check lists
- Monitoring during transport
- Safety during transport
- Context (i.e. aeromedical)
- Documentation and handover
- Insurance and indemnity

The Ambulance Response Programme

Ambulance response times vary according to clinical need (Table 3.1).
NHS England implemented new ambulance standards across the country in 2017 in order to[17]:
- Ensure that the sickest patients get the fastest response and that all patients get the right response first time.
- Support operational efficiency and performance
- Maintain a rapid response to the most seriously ill patients
- Reduce clinical risk in the ambulance system
- Improve quality of care for patients

TABLE 3.1 ■ Ambulance Response Targets

Category	Headline Description	Sub Description	Average Response Target	90th Percentile Response Target
1	Life threatening	A time critical life-threatening event requiring immediate intervention or resuscitation	7 min	15 min
2	Emergency	Potentially serious conditions that may require rapid assessment and urgent on-scene intervention and/or urgent transport	18 min	40 min
3	Urgent	An urgent problem (not immediately life threatening) that needs treatment to relieve suffering and transport or assessment and management at the scene with referral where needed within a clinically appropriate timeframe	None (mean indicator of 60 min)	2 h
4	Less urgent	Problems that are less urgent but require assessment and possibly transport within a clinically appropriate timeframe	None	3 h

From NHSE Ambulance Response Programme.

References

1. The King's Fund. *The quality of GP diagnosis and referral.* https://www.kingsfund.org.uk/sites/default/files/Diagnosis%20and%20referral.pdf. Accessed 24 May 2020.
2. Trimble M, Hamilton P. The thinking doctor: clinical decision making in contemporary medicine. *Clin Med.* 2016;16(4):343–346. https://doi.org/10.7861/clinmedicine.16-4-343.
3. Balla J, Heneghan C, Thompson M, et al. Clinical decision making in a high-risk primary care environment: a qualitative study in the UK. *BMJ Open.* 2012;2(1):e000414. https://doi.org/10.1136/bmjopen-2011-000414.
4. NHS Improvement. *Guide to Reducing Long Hospital Stays.* https://improvement.nhs.uk/documents/2898/Guide_to_reducing_long_hospital_stays_FINAL_v2.pdf. Accessed 24 May 2020.
5. NHS Improvement. *Rapid Improvement Guide to: The 6 As of Managing Emergency Admissions.* https://improvement.nhs.uk/documents/630/6As-managing-emergency-admissions-RIG.pdf. Accessed 24 May 2020.
6. The King's Fund. *Avoiding Hospital Admissions What Does the Research Evidence Say?* https://www.kingsfund.org.uk/sites/default/files/Avoiding-Hospital-Admissions-Sarah-Purdy-December2010_0.pdf. Accessed 24 May 2020.
7. NHSE. Mental Capacity Act. https://www.nhs.uk/conditions/social-care-and-support-guide/making-decisions-for-someone-else/mental-capacity-act/. Accessed 24 May 2020.
8. Department for Education, et al. *Safeguarding children.* https://www.gov.uk/topic/schools-colleges-childrens-services/safeguarding-children. Accessed 24 May 2020.
9. Office of the Public Guardian. *Safeguarding policy: protecting vulnerable adults.* https://www.gov.uk/government/publications/safeguarding-policy-protecting-vulnerable-adults. Accessed 24 May 2020.
10. Department of Health and Social Care. *Statutory guidance: care and support statutory guidance.* https://www.gov.uk/government/publications/care-act-statutory-guidance/care-and-support-statutory-guidance. Accessed 24 May 2020.
11. Home Office. *Channel guidance.* https://www.gov.uk/government/publications/channel-guidance. Accessed 24 May 2020.
12. Department of Health and Social Care. *Domestic abuse: a resource for health professionals.* https://www.gov.uk/government/publications/domestic-abuse-a-resource-for-health-professionals. Accessed 24 May 2020.
13. Public Health England. *Human Trafficking: Migrant Health Guide.* https://www.gov.uk/guidance/human-trafficking-migrant-health-guide. Accessed 24 May 2020.
14. National FGM. *Support clinics overview – female genital mutilation (FGM).* https://www.nhs.uk/conditions/female-genital-mutilation-fgm/. Accessed 24 May 2020.
15. Intercollegiate Board for Training in Pre-Hospital Emergency Medicine. *Sub-specialty training in pre-hospital emergency medicine: curriculum and assessment system.* http://www.ibtphem.org.uk/media/1039/sub-specialty-training-in-phem-curriculum-assessment-system-edition-2–2015.pdf. Accessed 24 May 2020.
16. The Faculty of Intensive Care Medicine and Society of Intensive. Care *Guidance on: the transfer of the critically Ill adult.* https://www.ficm.ac.uk/sites/default/files/transfer_critically_ill_adult_2019.pdf. Accessed 24 May 2020.
17. NHSE. Ambulance Response Programme. https://www.england.nhs.uk/urgent-emergency-care/improving-ambulance-services/arp/. Accessed 24 May 2020.
18. Potter PA, Perry AG, Stockert PA, Hall AM, Ostendorf WR. *Fundamentals of Nursing.* 9th ed. St. Louis: Elsevier; 2017:53.

Risk Management and Urgent Care Preparedness

Hazard and Risk

The human response to risk is contextual and has evolved over the ages[1]:

- The medieval perspective is when hazards (disease, violence, poverty) were ubiquitously involved in a perception of acceptance and helplessness with the evolution of belief systems to 'ward off' danger
- The modern approach involves increasing desires to control hazard and calculate risk with the belief that risk is a 'deviation' from the norm

  Implications of getting a risk assessment wrong may include:

- Clinical:
  - Safety incident or suboptimal outcome
  - Patient satisfaction
- Personal:
  - Stress
  - Inefficiency
- System:
  - Serious untoward incident (SUI)
  - Never event
  - Inefficiency
  - Financial

  Risk can be defined as 'the possibility of loss or injury' and is measured using the likelihood that harm or damage may occur and the consequence/severity of the outcome.

  Risk management in urgent care is:

- A systematic process to identify and control risks to the benefit of service users, staff and the public
- About improving quality and reducing harm

- Not confined to clinical practice, but also encompasses health and safety for clients, patients, visitors and staff, as well as environmental issues
- Not limited to physical injury but also includes financial damage and psychological harm Identification, assessment, treatment and monitoring of risk should always be considered:
- If new projects or services are undertaken
- When major changes are made or incidents occur
- On a regular basis (to include certain legal requirements, i.e. fire and health and safety policies)
- To support decision making by analysing risks and benefits of different courses of action
- With a view to being risk-aware, not risk-averse
- Using a risk scoring matrix such as that shown in Table 4.1.

Risk is related to the association between the consequence (or outcome) of an event and the likelihood that it will occur. Scores derived can inform a red/amber/green (RAG) rating that helps prioritise subsequent actions.

TABLE 4.1 ▏ **Risk Scoring Matrix**

		Likelihood				
		1	**2**	**3**	**4**	**5**
		Rare	**Unlikely**	**Possible**	**Likely**	**Almost Certain**
Consequence	1. Negligible	1	2	3	4	5
	2. Minor	2	4	6	8	10
	3. Moderate	3	6	9	12	15
	4. Major	4	8	12		
	5. Catastrophic	5	10			

Scores obtained from the risk matrix can then be assigned grades as follows:
1-6 – Low risk – Green
7-12 – Moderate risk – Amber
Over 12 – High risk – Red

Risk Management and System Design in the Context of Urgent Care

An overarching need exists for shared governance and whole system partnership working. Planning and delivery of urgent and emergency care improvements are divided between system resilience groups (SRGs) and Urgent and Emergency Care Networks (UECNs), with networks focussed on programmes that cannot easily be delivered at a more local level by SRGs or clinical commissioning groups (CCGs).

High-level considerations include:
- Clinical planning and patient flow
  - The National Health Service (NHS) Long Term Plan directs that urgent and emergency care services should be designed to produce a system that is safe, sustainable and that consistently provides high-quality care, with the intention that[2]:
    - Adults and children with urgent care needs should be looked after by a highly responsive service that delivers care as close to home as possible, minimising disruption and inconvenience for patients, carers and families
    - Those people with more serious or life-threatening emergency care needs, should be treated in centres with the right expertise, processes and facilities to maximise the prospects of survival and a good recovery
    - Capacity and demand (patterns and levels) should be understood
    - Imbalances between demand and capacity that create bottlenecks and delays should be avoided

- The need for higher-level risk management reducing variation in clinical practice between different parts of the system is with the logic that:
  - Unwarranted variation is a major obstacle to achieving safe, cost-effective patient care and flow
  - Simple rules should set boundaries within which health professionals and managers work
  - Urgent or emergency care patients in any setting should receive the earliest possible review by a senior clinical decision-maker
  - UUC systems should use appropriate triage/early warning scoring systems
  - People in mental health crisis should have their mental as well as any physical health needs assessed as rapidly as possible by an appropriate clinician
  - Activities should be prioritised to achieve the earliest possible discharge of patients
  - Frail older people and younger people with specific vulnerabilities should be assertively managed
  - Patients should be promptly assessed and placed into the most appropriate care stream to meet their needs
  - Continuity of patient care should be sought
  - Capacity should be designed to manage variation in demand, not just average demand
- Escalation plans
  - Local integrated health and social care escalation plans which clearly define trigger levels for escalation across all organisations
  - The practical and concrete actions taken by individual organisations in the event of escalation being triggered
  - Timely de-escalation protocols
  - Sufficient clinical leadership and involvement from primary and secondary care to resolve local issues in relation to escalation

Local (provider level) risks are commonplace and may include considerations such as:
- Clinical
  - Does this child need antibiotics?
  - Which patient needs to be seen next?
  - What may happen if these two drugs are prescribed together?
- System
  - How many nurse practitioners need to work in the unit on Christmas day?
  - Where should staff and capabilities (i.e. ambulances) be placed?

Learning From Significant Event Analysis and Serious Untoward Incidents

Definitions and threshold of SUIs[3]:
- SUIs are adverse events where the consequences to patients, families and carers, staff or organisations are so significant, or the potential for learning is so great, that a heightened level of response is justified
- Includes acts or omissions in care that result in: unexpected or avoidable death, unexpected or avoidable injury resulting in serious harm – including those where the injury required treatment to prevent death or serious harm, abuse, 'never events', incidents that prevent (or threaten to prevent) an organisation's ability to continue to deliver an acceptable quality of healthcare services and incidents that cause widespread public concern resulting in a loss of confidence in healthcare services
- They can extend beyond incidents that affect patients directly and include incidents which may indirectly impact patient safety or an organisation's ability to deliver ongoing healthcare

- They require investigation in order to identify the factors that contributed towards the incident occurring and the fundamental issues (or root causes) that underpinned these
- They can be isolated, single events or multiple linked or unlinked events signalling systemic failures within a commissioning or health system
  Serious incidents *must* be declared in the event of:
- Severe harm which includes chronic pain (continuous, long-term pain of more than 12 weeks or after the time that healing would have been thought to have occurred in pain after trauma or surgery)
- Psychological harm, impairment to sensory, motor or intellectual function or impairment to normal working or personal life, which is not likely to be temporary (i.e. has lasted, or is likely to last, for a continuous period of at least 28 days)
- Acts and/or omissions occurring as part of NHS-funded healthcare (including in the community) that result in unexpected or avoidable death of one or more people; this includes suicide/self-inflicted death and homicide by a person in receipt of mental healthcare within the recent past
- Unexpected or avoidable injury to one or more people that has resulted in serious harm
- Unexpected or avoidable injury to one or more people that requires further treatment by a healthcare professional in order to prevent the death of the service user or serious harm
- Actual or alleged abuse; sexual, physical or psychological abuse; or acts of omission which constitute neglect, exploitation, financial or material abuse, discriminative and organisational abuse, self-neglect, domestic abuse, human trafficking and modern-day slavery where healthcare did not take appropriate action/intervention to safeguard against such abuse occurring or where the abuse occurred during the provision of NHS-funded care
  When dealing with SUIs, the provider should consider:
- The needs of those affected should be the primary concern of those involved in the response and the investigation
- Patients and their families/carers and victims' families must be involved and supported throughout the investigation process
- Providers are responsible for the safety of their patients, visitors and others using their services and must ensure robust systems are in place for recognising, reporting, investigating and responding to serious incidents and for arranging and resourcing investigations
- Commissioners are accountable for quality assuring the robustness of their providers' Serious Incident investigations and the development and implementation of effective actions by the provider to prevent recurrence of similar incidents
- Investigations under this framework are not conducted to hold any individual or organisation to account, as there are other processes for that purpose, including criminal proceedings, disciplinary procedures, employment law and systems of service and professional regulation, such as the Care Quality Commission (CQC) and the Nursing and Midwifery Council, the Health and Care Professions Council, and the General Medical Council. Investigations should link to these other processes where appropriate
- They must be declared internally as soon as possible and immediate action must be taken to establish the facts; ensure the safety of the patient(s), service users and staff; and secure all relevant evidence to support further investigation
- They should be disclosed as soon as possible to the patient, their family (including victims' families where applicable) or carers
- The commissioner must be informed of a Serious Incident within two working days of it being discovered
- Other regulatory, statutory and advisory bodies, such as CQC, Monitor or NHS Trust Development Authority, must also be informed as appropriate without delay; discussions

should be held with other partners (including the police or local authority, for example) if other externally led investigations are being undertaken

- The recognised system-based method for conducting investigations, commonly known as root cause analysis (RCA), should be applied for the investigation of Serious Incidents
- They should be closed by the relevant commissioner when they are satisfied that the investigation report and action plan meet the required standard
'Never events' are:
- Defined as Serious Incidents, although not all never events necessarily result in serious harm or death
- An incident (or series of incidents) that prevents, or threatens to prevent, an organisation's ability to continue to deliver an acceptable quality of healthcare services, including (but not limited to) the following:
  - Caused or contributed to by weaknesses in care/service delivery (including lapses/acts and/ or omission) as opposed to a death which occurs as a direct result of the natural course of the patient's illness or underlying condition where this was managed in accordance with best practice
  - Includes those in receipt of care within the last 6 months, but this is a guide, and each case should be considered individually
  - May include failure to take a complete history, gather information from which to base care plan/treatment, assess mental capacity and/or seek consent to treatment, or fail to share information when to do so would be in the best interest of the client in an effort to prevent further abuse by a third party and/or to follow policy on safer recruitment
- Arise from failure of strong systemic protective barriers
- Can involve:
  - Failures in the security, integrity, accuracy or availability of information are often described as data loss and/or information governance-related issues
  - Property damage
  - Inappropriate enforcement/care under the Mental Health Act (1983) and the Mental Capacity Act (2005), including Mental Capacity Act, Deprivation of Liberty Safeguards (MCA DOLS)
  - Systematic failure to provide an acceptable standard of safe care
  - Major loss of confidence in the service, including prolonged adverse media coverage or public concern about the quality of healthcare or an organisation
A 'near miss':
- Can be classed as a serious incident because the outcome of an incident does not always reflect the potential severity of harm that could be caused should the incident (or a similar incident) occur again
- Is characterised by an assessment of risk that considers:
  - The likelihood of the incident occurring again if current systems/processes remain unchanged; and
  - The potential for harm to patients, staff and the organisation should the incident occur again

Principles of Emergency Preparedness, Response and Recovery

The NHS needs to plan for, and respond to, a wide range of incidents and emergencies that could affect health or patient care. These could range from extreme weather conditions to an outbreak of an infectious disease or a major transport accident. The Civil Contingencies Act

(2004) requires NHS organisations and providers of NHS-funded care to show that they can deal with such incidents while maintaining services. This programme of work is referred to in the health community as emergency preparedness, resilience and response (EPRR)

Relevant legislation:

- Civil Contingencies Act 2004
- Contingencies Planning Regulations 2005
- NHS Act 2006
  - Section 252 A
  - Emergency Planning
  - Statutory Guidance
  - Emergency Response and Recovery
  - Statutory Guidance
- Health and Social Care Act 2012
- NHS EPRR Framework 2013 Amended 2015

Categories of responders:

- Category 1 (primary responders)
  - Department of Health on behalf of Secretary of State for Health
  - NHS England
  - Acute service providers
  - Ambulance service providers
  - Public Health England (PHE)
  - Local authorities (Inc. Directors of Public Health [DsPH])
- Category 2 responders (supporting agencies)
  - CCGs
- Uncategorised Responders
  - Primary care, including out-of-hours providers
  - Community providers
  - Mental health service providers
  - Specialist providers

Category 1 responders' duties:

- Assess the risk of emergencies occurring and use this to inform contingency planning
- Put in place emergency plans
- Put in place business continuity management arrangements
- Put in place arrangements to make information available to the public about civil protection matters and maintain arrangements to warn, inform and advise the public in the event of an emergency
- Share information with other local responders to enhance co-ordination
- Cooperate with other local responders to enhance co-ordination and efficiency

Types of incident:

- Business continuity incident
  - An event or occurrence that disrupts, or might disrupt, an organisation's normal service delivery below acceptable predefined levels
  - Critical incident: any localised incident where the level of disruption results in the organisation temporarily or permanently losing its ability to deliver critical services, patients may have been harmed or the environment is not safe, requiring special measures and support from other agencies to restore normal operating functions.
  - Major incident: any occurrence that presents a serious threat to the health of the community or causes such numbers or types of casualties as to require special arrangements to be implemented (see next page)

'Anatomy' of an incident:
- Become aware of an undesired event
- Calls to 999
- Ambulance teams attend the scene
- Ambulance control creates a response strategy
- Notifies hospitals
- Declare major incident
- Treat casualties
- Restore normality
- Stand down activities
- Debrief

Advantages of declaring a major incident:
- Focuses the minds of staff
- Additional resources become available
- Comms team are involved
  - Warning and informing
- Security becomes involved (lockdown)
  - Dignity for friends and relatives
  - Press intrusions

Follow-on activities:
- Police evidence gathering
- Police casualty bureaux
- Dealing with friends and relatives
- Dealing with embassies
- Counselling
  - Patients
  - Friends and relatives
  - Staff (direct and indirect)

Post-incident:
- Hot debriefing
- Cold debriefing
- Lessons learnt
- Review of plans
- Training of new processes

The Role of Urgent Care Services in Relation to a Major Incident

A major incident is[4]:
- Any incident where the location, number, severity or type of live casualties requires extraordinary resources
- It is classified as:
  - Natural or man-made
  - Simple or compound
  - Compensated or uncompensated
- Most major incidents in developed countries are man-made, simple and compensated

Three distinct aspects to emergency preparedness are:
- Preparation
- Response
- Recovery

Management and support priorities are:

- Command
- Safety
- Communication
- Assessment
- Triage
- Treatment
- Transport

Major incident messages are:

- 'Major incident – standby': this alerts the hospital that a major incident is possible. A limited number of staff need to be informed
- 'Major incident declared – activate plan': in this case, the incident has occurred and a full response is required
- 'Major incident – cancelled'

First key information:

- **M** Major incident – Confirm call-sign. Advise major incident 'standby' or 'declared'
- **E** Exact location – Grid reference, road names, landmarks, etc.
- **T** Type of incident – Rail, chemical, road traffic collision, etc.
- **H** Hazards – Actual and potential
- **A** Access/egress – Safe direction to approach and depart
- **N** Number of casualties – An estimate in the first instance and then upgraded with their severity/type
- **E** Emergency services – Present and/or required

Management of Major Incident Situations

The roles and responsibilities of the Ambulance Service at a major incident include:

- Establishing a forward control point
- Saving life
- Preventing further injury
- Relieving suffering
- Liaising with other emergency services
- Determining the receiving hospitals
- Mobilising necessary additional medical resources
- Providing communications for health service resources at the scene
- Providing a casualty clearing station
- Providing the ambulance parking and loading points
- Determining priorities for treatment and evacuation using triage
- Arranging means of transporting the injured
- Documenting the movement of casualties

There are five levels of medical intervention at the scene:

- Triage
- Life-saving first aid
- Advanced life support
- Specialist medical support
- Packaging for transport

The roles and responsibilities of the mobile medical team at a major incident include:

- Primary triage at the site
- Treatment of live casualties at the site

- Secondary triage in the Casualty Clearing Station
- Treatment in the Casualty Clearing Station
- Triage for transport
- Treatment of casualties from other rescue services
- Assistance to a mobile surgical team if present
- Treatment of minor injuries at the scene
- Confirming death and labelling of the dead at the scene
  Large scale emergency planning should consider the following event scales:
- Major: individual hospitals handle the incident within current and long-established major incident plans. Number of casualties: tens
- Mass: larger-scale incident with the possibility of involving the closure or evacuation of a major health facility or persistent disruption over many days. Collective mutual aid response required from neighbouring trusts. Number of casualties: hundreds
- Catastrophic: an incident that is of such proportions that it severely disrupts health and social care and other support functions (e.g. water, electricity, transport). The required response exceeds local collective capacity. Number of casualties: thousands

The Psychological Needs of Those Involved in a Major Incident

The following groups are at risk of developing post-traumatic stress disorder (PTSD) following a major incident[5]:
- Victims
- Family members and friends of the victims
- People who witnessed the incidents
- Members of the public who were in the vicinity
- Those who attended to support as first responders
- Those who worked to provide subsequent care in hospital settings
  Lessons identified from the Westminster, London Bridge, Grenfell Tower and Finsbury Park incidents as well as more general research shows that[6]:
- Many individuals involved in a major incident (both as first responders and those who worked to provide subsequent care in hospital settings) are at risk of developing (typically short-term) mental health disorders
- In most cases, distress is transient and not associated with dysfunction or indicative of people developing mental disorders
- Some people's distress may last longer and is more incapacitating
- The majority of people do not require access to specialist mental healthcare; although a small proportion may do so
- It is important to access the right help at the right time. For example, providing a single session of debriefing as a form of treatment is not recommended
- Depending on the nature of events, around 70% or more of all people who are affected by major incidents are psychosocially resilient, despite their distress
- Distress reduces in severity if individuals receive the support they perceive as adequate, and intervening early can reduce the risks of people developing disorders later
- The majority of staff respond well and recover after emergencies if social support is available from relatives, friends and colleagues
- Employers should support staff by ensuring that they are well briefed, well-led and offered effective social and peer support
- Recent research shows that events encountered in emergency departments affect the psychosocial wellbeing of staff, and the cumulative effects may be negative and long-lasting

Key approaches to minimise the psychological impact should be:

- Acknowledge the importance of anticipated reactions (stress response) to a major incident
- Support people to develop and sustain their resilience; consider the important role of parents and carers or other trusted adults
- Utilise a multi-agency stepped model of care that provides a holistic continuum of care
- Ensure approaches are evidence-based and proportional, flexible and timely to respond to the emerging phased needs
- Provide clear and consistent messages and communication
- Ensure professionals and staff providing support have access to training, consultation and supervision

Phase one (initial) support should:

- Launch in reaction to the event
- Involve psychological first aid (PFA) and peer support
- Include the employer's leadership response to a major incident by communicating key messages of acknowledgement, self-care and support services, internal and external to the organisation
- Allow access to advice and support as necessary through existing universal services (community, primary care/GP and specialist services)
- Intervene using low-level interventions such as peer support, leaving biomedical mental healthcare for people who need it

Phase two (ongoing) support (weeks 2 to 4) should:

- Involve psychosocial support
- Aim to manage distress, but an emphasis on maintaining social connectedness
- Involve listening, advice and support
- Potentially refer some to a programme that offers monitoring over a longer period of time and access to screening

Phase three (additional) support (from 2 weeks onwards) should:

- Continue psychosocial support
- Monitor staff at risk via occupational health and possibly refer to:
  - Primary care
  - The trauma incident management (TRiM) service or equivalent
  - Specially created services to identify people who may need continuing support beyond 4 weeks
  - The Improving Access to Psychological Therapies (IAPT) service for more intensive psychosocial care

Phase four (specialist) support (when symptoms are still present between 4 and 12 weeks after an even) may be relevant for the following group who may be at higher risk of developing a mental disorder than the general population:

- Staff injured in the event or during the response
- Exposure to high severity of trauma
- Close proximity to the event
- Dissociative response during the event
- Significant (pre- or post-event) personal trauma, including developmental trauma and previous history of a mental disorder
- Personal or significant family psychiatric history
- Perceived absence of social support network
- Substance misuse
- Traumatic bereavement

Business Continuity Relevant to Urgent Care Services

A range of issues could interrupt business and clinical activity:
- Infrastructure:
  - Building damage
  - Fire, flooding
  - Loss of critical equipment – that is scanners, blood machines
- Logistics:
  - Loss of utilities/fuel
- Staff:
  - Sickness
  - Recruiting and retention crisis
- Information technology (IT):
  - Loss of capability
- Surges in demand:
  - Major incident
  - System escalation
  - Loss of neighbouring service

Business continuity plans might contain:
- A description of essential 'capability' and core services to be maintained
- Important communications/contacts list
- Risk assessments
- Actions on major incidents/system escalation
- Staff roles in an incident
- How to keep essential services functioning
- Initial action cards
- Key premises details
- Plans for a move to alternative premises

References

1. Lupton D. *Risk*. 2nd ed. London: Routledge; 2013.
2. NHSE. NHS Long Term Plan. https://www.longtermplan.nhs.uk. Accessed 24 May 2020.
3. NHSE. *Serious Incident Framework Supporting Learning to Prevent Recurrence.* https://www.england.nhs.uk/wp-content/uploads/2015/04/serious-incidnt-framwrk-upd.pdf. Accessed 20 May 2020.
4. Mackway-Jones K. *Major Incident Medical Management and Support: The Practical Approach at the Scene.* 2nd ed. London: BMJ Books; 2002.
5. NHSE. *London Mental Health Response to Major Incidents Pathway for Adult Witnesses.* https://www.healthylondon.org/wp-content/uploads/2017/10/London-incident-support-pathway-for-adult-witnesses.pdf. Accessed 24 May 2020.
6. NHSE. *Clinical Guidelines for Major Incidents and Mass Casualty Events.* https://www.england.nhs.uk/publication/clinical-guidelines-for-major-incidents-and-mass-casualty-events/. Accessed 20 May 2020.

Human Factors

Human Factors in Healthcare and Patient Safety

Several definitions of human factors in healthcare exist, such as:

- 'Enhancing clinical performance through an understanding of the effects of teamwork, tasks, equipment, workspace, culture and organisation on human behaviour and abilities and application of that knowledge in clinical settings'[1]
- 'Human factors encompass all those factors that can influence people and their behaviour. In a work context, human factors are the environmental, organisational and job factors, and individual characteristics which influence behaviour at work'[2]

   Human factors play a highly significant part in healthcare since[3]:

- They contribute directly to patient safety incidents
- Understanding them offers ways to minimise and mitigate human frailties, so reducing medical error and its consequences
- The system-wide adoption of these concepts offers a unique opportunity to support cultural change and empower the NHS to put patient safety and clinical excellence at its heart
- Their principles can be applied in the identification, assessment and management of patient safety risks, and in the analysis of incidents to identify learning and corrective actions
- Human factors understanding and techniques can be used to inform quality improvement in teams and services, support change management, and help to emphasise the importance of the design of equipment, processes and procedures
- The NHS must learn where it can from other high safety critical industries such as nuclear, petrochemical, military operations, rail, maritime, civil aviation and emergency services and thereby acknowledge that human factors is a way of thinking that should be incorporated as part of the design of processes, jobs and training

One well known example involves the case of Elaine Bromiley:[4]:

Case: Elaine Bromiley was a fit and healthy young woman who was admitted to hospital for routine sinus surgery. During the anaesthetic, she experienced breathing problems and the anaesthetist was unable to insert a device to secure her airway. After 10 minutes, it was a situation of 'can't intubate, can't ventilate'; a recognised anaesthetic emergency for which guidelines exist.

For a further 15 minutes, three highly experienced consultants made numerous unsuccessful attempts to secure Elaine's airway, and she suffered prolonged periods with dangerously low levels of oxygen in her bloodstream. Early on nurses informed the team that they had brought emergency equipment to the room and booked a bed in intensive care but neither were utilised.

Thirty-five minutes after the start of the anaesthetic it was decided that Elaine should be allowed to wake up naturally, and she was transferred to the recovery unit. When she failed to wake up, she was then transferred to the intensive care unit. Elaine never regained consciousness, and after 13 days, the decision was made to withdraw the ventilation support that was sustaining her life.

Investigation: It was found that every member of the team treating Elaine was experienced and technically highly competent, yet the series of events and actions still resulted in her death. Factors highlighted included:

■ Loss of situational awareness – the stress of the situation meant consultants involved became highly focused on repeated attempts to insert the breathing tube. As a result of this, they lost sight of the bigger picture, i.e. how long these attempts had been taking. This 'tunnel vision' meant they had no sense of time passing or the severity of the situation

■ Perception and cognition – actions were not in line with the emergency protocol. In the pressure of the moment, many options were being considered but they were not necessarily the options that made the most sense in hindsight

■ Teamwork – there was no clear leader. The consultants in the room were all providing help and support but no one person was seen to be in charge throughout. This led to a breakdown in the decision-making process and communication between the three consultants

■ Culture – nurses who sensed the urgency early on brought the emergency kit to the room, and then alerted the intensive care unit. They stated that these were available but did not raise their concerns aloud when they were not utilised. Other nurses who were aware of what was happening did not know how to broach the subject. The hierarchy of the team made assertiveness difficult despite the severity of the situation.

The fundamental basis of human factors relates to the issue of how human beings process information – we acquire information from the world around us, interpret and make sense of it and then respond to it. Errors can occur at each step in this process and contributing factors can include:

■ The misperceiving of situations despite the best of intentions is one of the main reasons that our decisions and actions can be flawed, resulting in making 'silly' mistakes – regardless of experience level, intelligence, motivation or vigilance

■ Problems with human–machine interactions (including equipment design) and human–human interactions such as communication, teamwork and organisational culture

■ Personal factors such as fatigue, stress, poor communication, distractions, physical demands and inadequate knowledge and skill mental workload[5]

The Swiss Cheese Model

James Reason's Swiss Cheese model (Fig. 5.1) is an established way of describing why organisational incidents occur.[6] It explains that good systems use defences, barriers and safeguards. Ideally, each is sound, but variations in each of them (the holes in the Swiss cheese) can sometimes align – when they do, then hazard can come into damaging contact with victims. Holes arise due to:

- Active failures – unsafe acts committed by people who are in direct contact with the patient or system (slips, lapses, fumbles, mistakes, procedural violations)
- Latent conditions – the inevitable 'resident pathogens' within the system arising from management and systems design which either translate into error provoking conditions (time pressure, understaffing, inadequate equipment, fatigue, inexperience) or long-lasting holes (untrustworthy alarms and indicators, unworkable procedures, design and construction deficiencies, etc.)

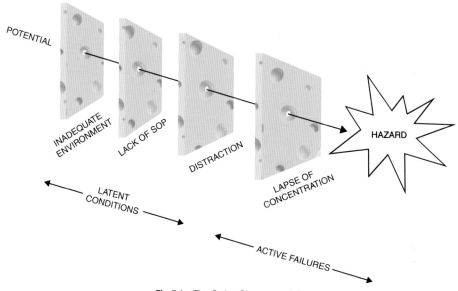

Fig. 5.1 The Swiss Cheese model.

The SHEEP Model

This model uses the acronym SHEEP (Fig. 5.2) to describe a human factors healthcare model.[7] Each of the elements listed has the potential to affect outcomes and clinical safety.

Systems:

- Informal (culture, information flow)
- Formal (information systems, organisational, information sets)

Human Interactions:

- Behaviours (interaction quality, communication quality)
- Task related (teams, lack of sense of time/situational awareness/options)
- Team dynamics and conflict (problems with leader/team/patient interaction/conflict)

Environment:

- Physical (temperature, lighting, noise, heat, size, etc.)
- Physical design (infrastructure, flow, accessibility, functional design)

ENVIRONMENT

HUMAN
INTERACTIONS   EQUIPMENT

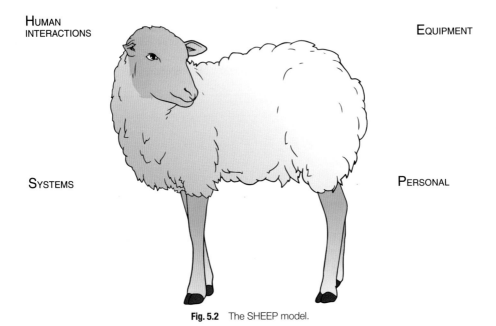

SYSTEMS   PERSONAL

Fig. 5.2   The SHEEP model.

- Dynamic interruptions (people, phones, bleeps, machines)
- Location change (complexity, distance)

Equipment:
- User interaction (training, skill, familiarity, preference, back up, ergonomics)
- Generic equipment problem (supply, storage, manufacturing, readiness, availability)
- Specific problems (failure, drugs – wing time/place/dose/patient)

Personal:
- External influences (time, pressure, time of day, shift patterns)
- Life events (commuting, parking, divorce, addiction)
- Values, attitudes, behaviours (mood, frustration, secure)
- Identity (race, gender, age)
- Physiological (tired, hungry, thirsty, stressed)

The WHO Surgical Safety Checklist

The WHO Surgical Safety checklist (Fig. 5.3) was developed after extensive consultation aiming to decrease errors and adverse events and increase teamwork and communication in surgery. The 19-item checklist has gone on to show significant reduction in both morbidity and mortality and is now used by a majority of surgical providers around the world.[8]

Surgical Safety Checklist

World Health Organization | Patient Safety
A World Alliance for Safer Health Care

Before induction of anaesthesia

(with at least nurse and anaesthetist)

Has the patient confirmed his/her identity, site, procedure, and consent?
☐ Yes

Is the site marked?
☐ Yes
☐ Not applicable

Is the anaesthesia machine and medication check complete?
☐ Yes

Is the pulse oximeter on the patient and functioning?
☐ Yes

Does the patient have a:

Known allergy?
☐ No
☐ Yes

Difficult airway or aspiration risk?
☐ No
☐ Yes, and equipment/assistance available

Risk of >500ml blood loss (7ml/kg in children)?
☐ No
☐ Yes, and two IVs/central access and fluids planned

Before skin incision

(with nurse, anaesthetist and surgeon)

☐ **Confirm all team members have introduced themselves by name and role.**

☐ **Confirm the patient's name, procedure, and where the incision will be made.**

Has antibiotic prophylaxis been given within the last 60 minutes?
☐ Yes
☐ Not applicable

Anticipated Critical Events

To Surgeon:
☐ What are the critical or non-routine steps?
☐ How long will the case take?
☐ What is the anticipated blood loss?

To Anaesthetist:
☐ Are there any patient-specific concerns?

To Nursing Team:
☐ Has sterility (including indicator results) been confirmed?
☐ Are there equipment issues or any concerns?

Is essential imaging displayed?
☐ Yes
☐ Not applicable

Before patient leaves operating room

(with nurse, anaesthetist and surgeon)

Nurse Verbally Confirms:
☐ The name of the procedure
☐ Completion of instrument, sponge and needle counts
☐ Specimen labelling (read specimen labels aloud, including patient name)
☐ Whether there are any equipment problems to be addressed

To Surgeon, Anaesthetist and Nurse:
☐ What are the key concerns for recovery and management of this patient?

This checklist is not intended to be comprehensive. Additions and modifications to fit local practice are encouraged.

Revised 1 / 2009

© WHO, 2009

Fig. 5.3 The WHO Surgical Safety Checklist. (World Health Organization, 2009.)

Crew Resource Management

The concept of crew resource management (CRM) initially developed from research performed in the aviation industry where factors to do with teamwork including hierarchy and communication are seen as important contributing factors to airline disasters.

An example of CRM issues contributing to an aviation disaster occurred on 22 December 1999, when the following incidents unfurled[9]:

- A Korean Air Cargo Flight (Boeing 747) crashed due to instrument malfunction and pilot error shortly after take-off from London Stansted Airport, killing all four crew on board. The captain was a highly experienced airman and former Colonel in the Republic of Korea Air Force. His junior officer was relatively very inexperienced
- The plane had taken off in darkness flown by the captain. When he tried to bank the plane to turn left, his instruments failed, depriving him of the opportunity to see how much bank he had applied. The junior officer's instruments were working – despite this and the fact that alarms began to sound, he failed to challenge his captain's actions or make any attempt to take over the flight with his own controls. An older and more experienced flight engineer did call out 'bank' four times in 19 seconds, but the captain ignored his warnings, continued to ignore the chiming alarm and made no verbal response. Ultimately the increasing angle of the bank caused the aircraft to descend and explode on impact with the ground

CRM factors have clear application to clinical systems, particularly with respect to[10]:

- Cooperation
- Leadership
- Workload management
- Situational awareness
- Decision-making

Processes to optimise CRM that can be readily applied to healthcare settings include:

- Peer monitoring
- Briefings
- Defining standard operating procedures and standards
- Recognition of fatigue as a factor in performance
- Regular 'check rides' in the form of assessment
- Blame-free reporting culture
- Use of checklists
- Application of the principle of a 'sterile cockpit' (referring to an environment free of unnecessary distractions, something which is most important when a critical or complex procedure is being carried out such as medication delivery)[11]
- Briefings before and after clinical activity
- Making actions proactive and generative, rather than solely reactive to adverse events
- Focusing on systems rather than individuals
- Examination of 'latent risk factors' that may result in adverse events

Good communication within CRM involves:

- Respect for each other's roles
- Direct eye contact
- Introducing each other
- Using non-judgemental words
- Putting safety before self-esteem

Cognitive Bias

Clinicians typically employ 'heuristic reasoning' involving mental shortcuts that allow problem solving quickly and efficiently. These assist in shortening decision-making time without constantly stopping to consider the implications and the next courses of action. While helpful in many situations, they can also lead to cognitive bias.

Cognitive bias is a *systematic error in thinking* that affects the decisions and judgements that people make. Some relate to memory (the way events are remembered may be biased for a number of reasons, leading to biased thinking and decision-making), others relate to problems with attention (since attention is a limited resource, people have to be selective about what they pay attention to in the world around them)

Multiple types and causes of cognitive bias exist, including[12]:

- Confirmation bias: favouring information that conforms to existing beliefs and discounting evidence that does not conform
- Availability heuristic: placing greater value on information that comes to mind quickly, giving greater credence to this information and tending to overestimate the probability and likelihood of similar things happening in the future, i.e. missing a pulmonary embolism prompts excessive future D-dimer investigations
- Halo effect: the overall impression of a person influences feeling and thinking about his or her character; especially applies to physical attractiveness influencing the rating of other qualities
- Self-serving bias: the tendency to blame external forces when bad things happen and give self-credit when good things happen
- Attentional bias: the tendency to pay attention to some things while simultaneously ignoring others
- Actor-observer bias: the tendency to attribute actions to external causes while attributing other people's behaviour to internal causes, i.e. attributing own high cholesterol level to genetics while considering others to have a high level due to poor diet
- Functional fixedness: the tendency to see objects as only working in a particular way, i.e. not realising a low-grade clinician has leadership skills
- Anchoring bias: the tendency to rely too heavily on the very first piece of information learnt
- Mis-information effect: the tendency for post-event information to interfere with the memory of the original event
- False consensus effect: the tendency to overestimate how much other people agree
- Optimism bias: leads to the expectation of suffering less from misfortune and being more likely to attain success
- The Dunning–Kruger effect: the belief of being smarter and more capable than reality and being unable to recognise own incompetence
- Base rate neglect: ignoring the underlying incident rates of conditions, i.e. performing an angiogram in a young woman with positive exercise stress test even though the 'base rate' is so low in this population that this result is more likely false positive than true positive
- Conjunction rule: the incorrect belief that the probability of multiple events being true is greater than a single event ('Occam's razor' – a simple and unifying explanation is statistically more likely than multiple unrelated explanations), i.e. thinking that a confused patient with hypoxia and deranged renal function has a subdural/pulmonary embolism/obstruction simultaneously rather than simple pneumonia
- Overconfidence: inflated opinion of diagnostic ability leading to subsequent error, i.e. trusting assessments such as auscultation for pneumonia more than is reasonable

- Search satisfying: ceasing to look for further information or alternative answers when the first plausible solution is found, i.e. treating obvious pneumonia in an acutely dyspnoeic patient, then stopping investigations and failing to search for and recognise the secondary myocardial infarction
- Diagnostic momentum: continuing a clinical course of action instigated by previous clinicians without considering the information available and changing the plan if required (particularly if plan commenced by more senior clinician)
- The framing effect: reacting to a particular choice differently depending on how the information is presented

Ways of minimising bias include[13]:
- Bias-specific teaching
- Slowing down and reducing work intensity and pressure
- 'Meta-cognition' – the awareness of, and insight into one's own thought processes and consciously asking 'what else could this be?' or experimentally considering the 'opposite'
- Checklists – cognitive forcing tools that demand the user think in a more ordered fashion
- Teaching statistical principles
- Novel methods – assuming the first estimate to a quantitative answer is incorrect and attempting to answer again – the average of two answers is demonstrably more accurate (i.e. bedside weight estimation estimating a patient's weight at the bedside, or their baseline renal function when no historical measurements are available)
- Consider what data are truly relevant

Decision-Making in Urgent Medical Care

Decisions can be considered to have their own attributes[14]:
- Uniqueness: the extent to which the features of the decision are unlike others
- Certainty: the amount of information and clear guidelines that exist as to the interpretation of data and to guide a course of action
- Importance/criticalness/value conflict: the significance of the decision in relation to outcome and effects of negative consequences
- Stability – The extent and rate at which the environment surrounding the decision is changing or evolving, i.e. an unstable decision environment is where the patient's medical condition is changing at the time the decision is changing such that new data are being received and interpreted requiring a dynamic decision-making process
- Urgency: the extent to which an immediate decision needs to be made or whether it can be delayed
- Familiarity: the extent to which the decision being made is similar to decisions made in the past
- Congruence/conflict: the extent to which elements of the decision such as the inputs, goals, and environment of the decision fit, match and correspond with each other
- Number of variables: the amount of data that need to be considered and interpreted in order to make a decision
- Relevance of variables: the extent to which the data available contain information relevant to the decision being made that needs to be sorted from irrelevant material
- Risk: the estimation of the chance of an adverse or negative outcome occurring as a result of the decision

Numerous models exist to explain and describe clinical decision-making. Often, a clinician looks to seek 'an explanation of a particular fact by finding some salient features of the particular that allow it to be explained by some more general causative principles'. As examples[15]:

Deduction is reasoning from the general to the particular, i.e.:
- All the marbles in the jar are white
- These marbles are from the jar

- Therefore, these marbles must be white

Induction is reasoning from the particular to the general, i.e.:

- These marbles have come from the jar
- These marbles are white
- Therefore, the marbles in the jar are white

Abduction is more of an inference, an informed guess that fits with the known facts, i.e.:

- The marbles in the jar are white
- These marbles are white
- Therefore, these marbles have come from the jar

'Heuristics' involve more informal problem-solving methods, such as trial and error, that lead quickly to solutions. Senior clinicians are seldom conscious of the heuristic cognitive pathways they use to make decisions. Typical decision-making approaches include:

- Pattern recognition
- Scientific method: start with problem, develop a hypothesis, collect and analyse data, confirm or reject hypothesis
- Probabilities
- Differential diagnoses
- Investigations
- Treatment thresholds

The 'hypothetico-deductive' model involves:

- Information gathering
- Hypothesis generation:
  - Pattern recognition – occurring early, i.e. 'headache with neck stiffness and photophobia', which then changes slightly with the term 'thunderclap onset'
  - Ruling out worst case scenarios – ask questions to exclude significant differential diagnoses (i.e. for patients with chest pain) without confirming a definite diagnosis
  - Casablanca strategy – to 'round up the usual suspects' (akin to working on autopilot)
- Hypothesis testing
- Reflection

'Dual process theory' suggests that clinicians process information in two ways, termed System 1 and System 2:

- System 1 processing is 'intuitive, automatic, fast, efficient and effortless', involving the construction of mental maps and patterns, shortcuts and rules of thumb (heuristics) and 'mind-lines' (collectively reinforced, internalised tacit guidelines); these are developed through experience and repetition, usually based on early teaching, brief written summaries, seeing what other people do, talking to local colleagues and personal experience
- System 2 processing involves a careful, rational analysis and evaluation of the available information. It is effortful and time consuming
- Clinicians prefer to use System 1 processing whenever possible
- Neither System 1 nor System 2 are 'good' or 'bad'; System 1 decision-making can provide life-saving decisions very quickly, whereas System 2 decision-making can locate information that enables a decision to be made when System 1 is incapable of doing so
- System 2 processing takes more time, and this may not always be consistent with the pace required in clinical practice
- Gaps between evidence and practice may occur when a clinician develops a pattern of knowledge, which is then relied on for decisions using System 1 processing, without the activation of a System 2 check
- It is important for clinicians to identify when they should convert to System 2 thinking to make sure an important outcome is achieved or avoided

Regardless of the methodology behind it, a good clinical decision making requires a combination of experience and skills.[16] These skills include:

- Pattern recognition: learning from experience
- Critical thinking: removing emotion from our reasoning, being 'sceptical', with the ability to clarify goals, examine assumptions, be open-minded, recognise personal attitudes and bias, able to evaluate evidence
- Communication skills: active listening – the ability to listen to the patient, what they say - what they don't say, their story, their experiences and their wishes, thus enabling a patient-centred approach that embraces self-management; information provision – the ability to provide information in a comprehensible way to allow patients/clients, their carers and family to be involved in the decision-making process
- Evidence-based approaches: using available evidence and best practice guidelines as part of the decision-making process
- Teamwork: using the gathered evidence to enlist help, support and advice from colleagues and the wider multi-disciplinary team. It is important to liaise with colleagues, listen and be respectful, while also being persistent when you need support so that you can plan as a team when necessary
- Sharing: your learning and getting feedback from colleagues on your decision-making
- Reflection: using feedback from others, and the outcomes of the decisions to reflect on the decisions that were taken in order to enhance practice delivery in the future. It is also important to reflect on your whole decision-making strategies to ensure that you hone your decision-making skills and learn from experience

Communication Within and Between Teams

Communication and collaboration in health care is defined as health care professionals assuming complementary roles and cooperatively working together, sharing responsibility for problem-solving and making decisions to formulate and carry out plans for patient care.[17]

Effective communication within clinical teams is critical because[18]:

- Patients are likely to receive care from multiple individuals
- Ineffective communication is a leading cause of inadvertent patient harm
- Ineffective team communication leads to duplication of tests and delays in identification and treatment of deteriorating patients
- Communication deficits are especially common at the interface between primary and secondary care
- They can culminate in adverse events, including an increase in preventable hospital admissions
- Effective communication improves job satisfaction, increases staff retention and facilitates a culture of support and trust
- When individuals have confidence that their opinions will be heard, they are more likely to speak up

Barriers to effective teamworking and communication include:

- Inter-professional communication: professional groups have historically been trained to communicate in different ways, for example, doctors have traditionally had a more succinct approach to communication with an emphasis on facts, while nurses have had a more holistic focus
- Fear of failure: there is a culture embedded within healthcare, where mistakes are too often viewed as a personal failure

- Human factors, stress and fatigue: healthcare professionals operate in times of increasing stress and workload
- Team instability: shift work, and the changing delivery of healthcare, results in dynamic teams with constantly changing members and therefore a lack of stability and more handover of care than before
- Inconsistent technology: technology can enhance communication, but the NHS has not reached consistency in the use of technology between healthcare teams; increased focus on shared technology systems, including patient record sharing between primary and secondary care, should enhance communication between teams
- Hierarchy
  Organisational processes to improve communication may include:
- Team brief and debrief: to include consideration like:
  - Who is on the team?
  - Do all members understand and agree goals?
  - Are roles and responsibilities understood? What is our plan of care?
  - What is the availability of staff during the shift? How will workload be shared?
  - What resources are available
- SBAR: see Table 5.1
- Call-out and check-back: used to communicate critical information in an emergency; the clinician calls out questions and commands, ensuring that all team members are simultaneously informed of updates and can anticipate the next steps. Check-back is where confirmation is sought that information given by the sender is received and understood
- Two-challenge rule; designed to empower all team members to 'stop' an activity if they sense a safety concern. The first challenge should be in the form of a question, the second challenge should provide some support for the team member's concern. The team member challenged must acknowledge the concerns. If this does not result in a change, then the person with the concern should take stronger action, this may be talking to a supervisor or the next person up the chain of command
- Critical language: a mechanism to overcome the hierarchical nature of medicine ivy adopting the use of critical language – CUS stands for 'I'm Concerned, I'm Uncomfortable, this is unSafe', and is a three-step process that provides clarity, ensures that everyone stops and listens and is alerted to the seriousness of the situation; used only for serious and urgent issues, where the concern is significant
- Checklists and read-back protocols: outline the criteria for consideration in a particular process such as the WHO Surgical Safety checklist
- Huddles: complementary to briefs and debriefs, huddles occur part way through a shift or team task. Team members come together to review activity, allowing re-establishment of situational awareness
- Handover: with the introduction of more shift pattern working, communication during handover is more essential than ever. Handovers should include:
- Adequate time without interruptions
- Clear leadership throughout
- Exchange of sufficient and relevant information
- Discussion around clinically unstable and unwell patients, with clear and unambiguous plans
- Description and assignment of uncompleted tasks

The SBAR communication tool (situation, background, assessment, recommendation) was originally developed by the United States military for communication on nuclear submarines but has been successfully used in many different healthcare settings, particularly relating to improving

TABLE 5.1 ■ The SBAR Communication Tool – An Example of a Handover in an Urgent Treatment Centre

Situation	I have just triaged Mrs Jones and I am bringing her to you in the observation bay. Her observations are:

BP	96/66 mm Hg
Heart rate	118 bpm
SpO$_2$	90%
Temperature	39°C
Respiratory rate°	29 bpm

Background	Mrs Jones is a 68-year-old lady known to have chronic obstructive pulmonary disease (COPD). She has been unwell for the last five days with increasing cough and shortness of breath. Today she feels terrible.
Assessment	Mrs Jones seems to have an exacerbation of her COPD and I am worried she may have sepsis.
Recommendations	Please admit her to the bay and immediately repeat her observations and undertake a full clinical assessment. Please start our sepsis protocol and take the usual bloods including FBC, CRP and lactate. She is likely to need a P1 transfer to the hospital but do not delay starting treatment.

patient safety.[19] It allows staff to communicate assertively and effectively, reducing the need for repetition and the likelihood for errors. As the structure is shared, it also helps staff anticipate the information needed by colleagues and encourages assessment skills.

Teamworking

Successful teamworking depends upon[20]:

- Open communication
- Non-punitive environment
- Clear direction
- Clear and known roles and tasks for team members
- Respectful atmosphere
- Shared responsibility for team success
- Appropriate balance of member participation for the task at hand
- Acknowledgement and processing of conflict
- Clear specifications regarding authority and accountability
- Clear and known decision-making procedures
- Regular and routine communication and information sharing
- Enabling environment, including access to needed resources
- Mechanism to evaluate outcomes and adjust accordingly
- Design of systems to absorb errors through redundancy, standardisation, and checklists
- Movement from placing blame to designing safe processes and procedures, i.e. applying a systems approach

- Assurance of full immunity while implementing a non-punitive approach
- Debriefing of all events, including near misses, that have learning potential
- Introducing a permanent programme for risk identification, analysis and dissemination of the lessons learnt throughout the professional community
  Common barriers to inter-professional communication and collaboration include:
- Personal values and expectations
- Personality differences
- Hierarchy
- Disruptive behaviour
- Culture and ethnicity
- Generational differences
- Gender
- Historical inter-professional and intra-professional rivalries
- Differences in language and jargon
- Differences in schedules and professional routines
- Varying levels of preparation, qualifications and status
- Differences in requirements, regulations, and norms of professional education
- Fears of diluted professional identity
- Differences in accountability, payment and rewards
- Concerns regarding clinical responsibility
- Complexity of care
- Emphasis on rapid decision-making

Leadership

Leadership is:
- 'The transfer of emotion'
- Visionary
- Creative
- Inspirational
- Energising
- Transformational…
  Whereas management is:
- Day-to-day routine
- Transactional
- Requiring operational skills
- Steady-state
  The NHS Healthcare Leadership model describes nine dimensions of leadership behaviour[21]:
- Inspiring shared purpose:
  - Valuing a service ethos
  - Curious about how to improve services and patient care
  - Behaving in a way that reflects the principles and values of the NHS
- Leading with care
  - Having the essential personal qualities for leaders in health and social care
  - Understanding the unique qualities and needs of a team
  - Providing a caring, safe environment to enable everyone to do their jobs effectively
- Evaluating information
  - Seeking out varied information
  - Using information to generate new ideas and make effective plans for improvement or change

- Making evidence-based decisions that respect different perspectives and meet the needs of all service users
- Connecting our service
  - Understanding how health and social care services fit together and how different people, teams or organisations interconnect and interact
- Sharing the vision
  - Communicating a compelling and credible vision of the future in a way that makes it feel achievable and exciting
- Engaging the team
  - Involving individuals and demonstrating that their contributions and ideas are valued and important for delivering outcomes and continuous improvements to the service
- Holding to account
  - Agreeing clear performance goals and quality indicators
  - Supporting individuals and teams to take responsibility for results
  - Providing balanced feedback
- Developing capability
  - Building capability to enable people to meet future challenges
  - Using a range of experiences as a vehicle for individual and organisational learning
  - Acting as a role model for personal development
- Influencing for results
  - Deciding how to have a positive impact on other people
  - Building relationships to recognise other people's passions and concerns
  - Using interpersonal and organisational understanding to persuade and build collaboration

Various models or theories exist to describe the concept of 'leadership':

- Trait theory: particular traits and qualities are born or bred and rise to the top, particularly in challenging circumstances
- Functional theory: leadership is a 'job' that can be learnt and developed
- 'Style' approaches: in which it is the leader's 'influence' that is important – the leader informs subordinates what the important priorities are, then abdicate responsibility to subordinates
- Contingency theories: different leaders would excel in different sets of circumstances, or better leaders would change according to circumstances around them
- Transactional versus transformational
  - Transactional: a 'bargain' is struck between leaders and subordinates who are clear about the rewards that can be expected for certain actions or behaviours
  - Transformational: leaders present visions of new possibilities and individuals rising to the challenge through which they can both improve and fulfil themselves
  - Dialogical: the leader creates a landscape of possibilities while it remains clear what everyone's obligations and responsibilities are. the leader is not always in control but also sometimes a listener or servant – 'serve to lead'
  - Leadership and distribution – helps articulate how at an organisational level, use influence and how influence is seen as part of work practice and the development of talent

The NHS increasingly favours the concept of 'compassionate leadership', in which everyone in the workplace – 'from ward to board' – contributes to creating a climate of compassion for both staff and patients, drawing on the indisputable links that have been proven to exist between the experience of patients and the experience of staff.[22]

Key to compassionate leadership and the demonstration of compassion in clinical practice is the concept of emotional intelligence (EI) – 'the ability to monitor one's own and other people's emotions, to discriminate between different emotions and label them appropriately, and to use emotional information to guide thinking and behaviour'.[23,24]

Emotional Intelligence is explained by different models[25]:

The 'ability' model conceptualises EI as a standard intelligence or a group of mental traits or abilities that can be assessed with performance tests

The alternative 'mixed models' are the mixture of multiple constructs that include personality traits, personal competencies (e.g. optimism, self-esteem), self-awareness. self-regulation, social skills, empathy and motivation.

Bad Leadership

'Abusive' leadership:

- Engaging in aggressive or punitive behaviours towards employees
- Links to work place harassment, emotional abuse, bullying
  Passive leadership:
- Includes 'laissez-faire' and management by exception
- Intervene late
  Pseudo-transformational leadership:
- Individuals have elements of transformational leadership style but are self-interested rather than altruistic
- Promotes fear, obedience and dependence
  Toxic leadership:
- Autocratic
- Abuses position and authority to impose will
- Focused on maintaining tight control and intolerant of mistakes, falsely assuming that the same mistake would not happen to them
- This, coupled with a lack of trust in their subordinates, means that they don't delegate. Communication tends to be directive and top-down rather than 'two-way'
- Self-serving; they do not care about the organisation or the people within it
- Motivated by personal ambition

Managing Fatigue and Stress

Fatigue is a decline in mental and/or physical performance that results from prolonged exertion, sleep loss and/or disruption of the internal clock. It is highly important in healthcare because it is directly related to[26]:

- Patient safety
- Accidents
- Injuries
- Ill health
- Slower reactions
- Reduced ability to process information
- Memory lapses
- Absent-mindedness
- Decreased awareness
- Lack of attention
- Underestimation of risk, reduced coordination
- Reduced productivity
  Many factors contribute to fatigue:
- Poorly designed shift-working arrangements

- Long working hours that do not balance the demands of work with time for rest and recovery
- Prolonged physical activity
- Sleep loss and/or disruption of the internal clock
- Workload
- Type of work – machine-paced, complex or monotonous
  Particular considerations exist for managers:
- Fatigue needs to be managed – like any other hazard
- Legal duty is on employers to manage risks from fatigue – irrespective of any individual's willingness to work extra hours or preference for certain shift patterns for social reasons
- Compliance with the working time regulations alone is insufficient to manage the risks of fatigue
- Policies should be developed that specifically address and set limits on working hours, overtime and shift-swapping, and which guards against fatigue
- Policies must be both implemented, monitored and enforced – which may include developing a robust system of recording working hours, overtime, shift-swapping and on-call working
- Problems with overtime and shift-swapping may indicate inadequate resource allocation and staffing levels
- Sleep disturbances can lead to a 'sleep debt' and fatigue
- Night workers are particularly at risk of fatigue because their day sleep is often lighter, shorter and more easily disturbed because of daytime noise and a natural reluctance to sleep during daylight

Error Investigation and Management

Serious incidents in health care[27]:
- Also see Chapter 4
- Definition: 'Adverse events, where the consequences to patients, families and carers, staff or organisations are so significant or the potential for learning is so great, that a heightened level of response is justified'
- Include acts or omissions in care that result in; unexpected or avoidable death, unexpected or avoidable injury resulting in serious harm - including those where the injury required treatment to prevent death or serious harm, abuse, 'never events', incidents that prevent (or threaten to prevent) an organisation's ability to continue to deliver an acceptable quality of healthcare services and incidents that cause widespread public concern resulting in a loss of confidence in healthcare services
- Must be declared internally as soon as possible and immediate action must be taken to establish the facts, ensure the safety of the patient(s), other services users and staff, and to secure all relevant evidence to support further investigation
- Should be disclosed as soon as possible to the patient, their family (including victims' families where applicable) or carers
- The commissioner must be informed of a Serious Incident within 2 working days of it being discovered
- Other regulatory, statutory and advisory bodies, such as care quality commission (CQC), Monitor or NHS Trust Development Authority, must also be informed as appropriate without delay
- Examples of serious incidents in the NHS include:
  - Unexpected or avoidable death of one or more people
  - Unexpected or avoidable injury to one or more people that has resulted in serious harm
  - Unexpected or avoidable injury to one or more people that requires further treatment by a healthcare professional in order to prevent death or serious harm

- Actual or alleged abuse; sexual abuse, physical or psychological ill-treatment, or acts of omission which constitute neglect, exploitation, financial or material abuse, discriminative and organisational abuse, self-neglect, domestic abuse, human trafficking and modern-day slavery where:
  - Healthcare did not take appropriate action/intervention to safeguard against such abuse occurring
  - Where abuse occurred during the provision of NHS-funded care
- Never events
- An incident (or series of incidents) that prevents, or threatens to prevent, an organisation's ability to continue to deliver an acceptable quality of healthcare services
- Major loss of confidence in the service, including prolonged adverse media coverage or public concern about the quality of healthcare or an organisation

Serious incidents may be identified through various routes including:

- Incidents identified during the provision of healthcare by a provider, for example, patient safety incidents or serious/distressing/catastrophic outcomes for those involved
- Allegations made against or concerns expressed about a provider by a patient or third party
- Initiation of other investigations, for example: Serious Case Reviews (SCRs), Safeguarding Adult Reviews (SARs), Safeguarding Adults Enquires
- Information shared at quality surveillance group meetings
- Complaints
- Whistle blowing
- Prevention of Future Death reports issued by the coroner

Managing, investigating and learning from serious incidents requires a considerable amount of time and resource and should include:

- Prioritising
- Opportunities for investing time in learning (root cause analysis)
- Prevalence/recording

Root Cause Analysis

The CQC has highlighted five opportunities for improvement[28]:

- Prioritise serious incidents that require full investigation and develop alternative methods for managing and learning from other types of incident
- Routinely involve patients and families in investigations
- Engage and support the staff involved in the incident and investigation process
- Use skilled analysis to move the focus of investigation from the acts or omissions of staff, to identifying the underlying causes of the incident
- Use human factors principles to develop solutions that reduce the risk of the same incidents happening again.

Root cause analysis (RCA) aims to define the 'deepest' significant contribution to error and significant incidents[29]:

- The 'Five Whys' approach was devised by Toyota as they developed their manufacturing methodologies
- It can assist in formalising and describing a problem, using brainstorming to ask why the problem occurs, then drilling down until the ultimate source is identified, i.e.:
  - The patient was late in theatre, it caused a delay
  - Why?…There was a long wait for a trolley
  - Why?…A replacement trolley had to be found
  - Why?…The original trolley's safety rail was worn and had eventually broken
  - Why?…It had not been regularly checked for wear

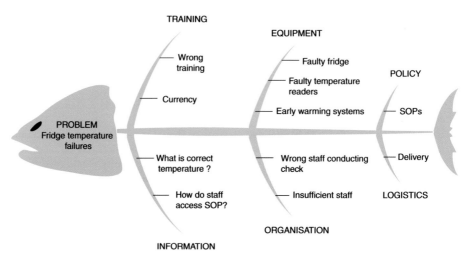

Fig. 5.4 Cause and effect (Fishbone) analysis – example assessing continued fridge temperature failures.

- Outcome: The root cause here is that there is no equipment maintenance schedule; setting up a proper maintenance schedule helps ensure that patients are not late due to faulty equipment

Once the root cause has been identified it may be useful to complete a cause and effect (fishbone) analysis (Fig. 5.4).[30]

Some point out limitations of RCA in that[31]:

- It is a promising incident investigation technique borrowed from other high-risk industries, but has failed to live up to its potential in healthcare
- A key problem with RCA is its name, which implies a singular, linear cause
- Other problems include the questionable quality of many RCAs, their susceptibility to political hijack, their tendency to produce poor risk controls, poorly functioning feedback loops, failure to aggregate learning across incidents and confusion about blame and responsibility
- Implementation and evaluation of risk controls to eliminate or minimise identified hazards need to become a more visible feature of the RCA process
- To maximise learning, lessons learnt from incidents, descriptions of implemented risk controls and their effectiveness need to be shared within and across organisations

Regardless of the cause of an error or adverse event, it remains important to support clinicians who may feel guilt, fear, anxiety or anger and may doubt themselves, experience social withdrawal, disturbing and troubling memories and depression and fear peer judgement.[32]

References

1. National Quality Board. *Human Factors in Healthcare: A Concordat From the National Quality Board*. https://www.england.nhs.uk/wp-content/uploads/2013/11/nqb-hum-fact-concord.pdf. Accessed 20 May 2020.
2. Patient Safety First. *The 'How to Guide' for Implementing Human Factors in Healthcare*. https://www.guysand-stthomas.nhs.uk/resources/education-training/sail/reading/human-factors.pdf. Accessed 24 May 2020.
3. National Quality Board. Human factors in healthcare. http://www.england.nhs.uk/ourwork/part-rel/nqb/ag-min/. Accessed 24 May 2020.

4. FutureLearn. *The Story of Elaine Bromiley.* https://www.futurelearn.com/info/courses/airway-matters/0/steps/68647. Accessed 10 August 22.

5. Health and Safety Executive. Human factors: fatigue. https://www.hse.gov.uk/humanfactors/topics/fatigue.htm. Accessed 24 May 2020.

6. Reason J. *Human Error: Models and Management.* British Medical Journal Publishing Group; 2000.

7. McCaig R. Human factors in healthcare: level one. *Occup Med.* 2014;64(7):563. https://doi.org/10.1093/occmed/kqu131.

8. World Health Organisation. *WHO Surgical Safety Checklist.* https://www.who.int/patientsafety/safesurgery/checklist/en/. Accessed 24 May 2020.

9. Aviation Accidents. *CRM.* http://www.aviation-accidents.net/tag/crm/page/3/. Accessed 24 May 2020.

10. Seager L, Smith DW, Patel A, et al. Applying aviation factors to oral and maxillofacial surgery – the human element. *Br J Oral Maxillofac Surg.* 2013;51(1):8–13. https://doi.org/10.1016/j.bjoms.2011.11.024.

11. Wadhera RK, Parker SH, Burkhart HM, et al. Is the 'sterile cockpit' concept applicable to cardiovascular surgery critical intervals or critical events? The impact of protocol-driven communication during cardiopulmonary bypass. *J Thorac Cardiovasc Surg.* 2010;139(2):312–319. https://doi.org/10.1016/j.jtcvs.2009.10.048.

12. O'Sullivan E, Schofield SJ. Cognitive bias in clinical medicine. *J R Coll Physicians Edinb.* 2018;48(3):225–232. https://doi.org/10.4997/JRCPE.2018.306.

13. Klein JG. *Five Pitfalls in Decisions About Diagnosis and Prescribing.* British Medical Journal Publishing Group; 2005.

14. Smith M, Higgs J, Ellis E. *Factors Influencing Clinical Decision Making. Clinical Reasoning in the Health Professions.* 3rd ed. 8th (section 2) ed. Sydney: Butterworth-Heinemann; 2008:89–100.

15. Rapezzi C, Ferrari R, Branzi A. *White Coats and Fingerprints: Diagnostic Reasoning in Medicine and Investigative Methods of Fictional Detectives.* British Medical Journal Publishing Group; 2005.

16. NHS: Education for Scotland. *Clinical Decision Making.* http://www.effectivepractitioner.nes.scot.nhs.uk/media/254840/clinical%20decision%20making.pdf. Accessed 24 May 2020.

17. Donald F, Mohide EA, DiCenso A, et al. Nurse practitioner and physician collaboration in long-term care homes: survey results. *Can J Aging.* 2009;28(1):77–87. https://doi.org/10.1017/S0714980809090060.

18. Royal College of Physicians. Improving teams in healthcare. https://www.rcplondon.ac.uk/projects/improving-teams-healthcare. Accessed 24 May 2020.

19. NHS Improvement. *SBAR Communication Tool.* https://www.england.nhs.uk/wp-content/uploads/2021/03/qsir-sbar-communication-tool.pdf. Accessed 24 May 2020.

20. Hughes R. *Patient Safety and Quality: An Evidence-Based Handbook for Nurses.* Rockville, MD: Agency for Healthcare Research and Quality (US); 2008.

21. NHS Leadership Academy. *Healthcare Leadership Model: The Nine Dimensions of Leadership Behaviour.* https://www.leadershipacademy.nhs.uk/wp-content/uploads/2014/10/NHSLeadership-LeadershipModel-colour.pdf. Accessed 24 May 2020.

22. NHSE. *Building and Strengthening Leadership: Leading With Compassion.* https://www.england.nhs.uk/wp-content/uploads/2014/12/london-nursing-accessible.pdf. Accessed 24 May 2020.

23. del Carmen MDC, Valero-Moreno S, Prado-Gascó VJ. Evaluation of emotional skills in nursing using regression and QCA models: a transversal study. *Nurse Educ Today.* 2019;74:31–37. https://doi.org/10.1016/j.nedt.2018.11.019.

24. Nightingale S, Spiby H, Sheen K, et al. The impact of emotional intelligence in health care professionals on caring behaviour towards patients in clinical and long-term care settings: findings from an integrative review. *Int J Nurs Stud.* 2018;80:106–117. https://doi.org/10.1016/j.ijnurstu.2018.01.006.

25. Vandewaa E, Turnipseed D, Cain G. Panacea or placebo? an evaluation of emotional intelligence in healthcare workers. *J Health Hum Serv Adm.* 2016;38(4):438–477.

26. Health and Safety Executive. *Human Factors: Fatigue.* https://www.hse.gov.uk/humanfactors/topics/fatigue.htm. Accessed 25 October 2020.

27. NHSE. *Serious Incident Framework Supporting Learning to Prevent Recurrence.* https://www.england.nhs.uk/wp-content/uploads/2015/04/serious-incidnt-framwrk-upd.pdf. Accessed 24 May 2020.

28. Care Quality Commission. *Briefing: Learning From Serious Incidents in NHS Acute Hospitals: A Review of the Quality of Investigation Reports.* https://www.cqc.org.uk/sites/default/files/20160608_learning_from_harm_briefing_paper.pdf. Accessed 24 May 2020.

29. NHS Improvement. *Root Cause Analysis Using Five Whys*. https://www.england.nhs.uk/wp-content/uploads/2022/02/qsir-using-five-whys-to-review-a-simple-problem.pdf. Accessed 20 May 2020.

30. NHS Improvement. *Cause and Effect (Fishbone)*. https://www.england.nhs.uk/wp-content/uploads/2021/12/qsir-cause-and-effect-fishbone.pdf. Accessed 24 May 2020.

31. Peerally MF, Carr S, Waring J, et al. The problem with root cause analysis. *BMJ Qual Saf*. 2017;26(5):417–422. https://doi.org/10.1136/bmjqs-2016-005511.

32. Edrees H, Federico F. *Supporting Clinicians After Medical Error*. British Medical Journal Publishing Group; 2015.

Operational Performance

Local and National Operational Guidance

The National Health Service (NHS) responds to more than 110 million urgent calls or visits every year and has developed an overarching national service specification for the provision of a functionally integrated 24/7 urgent care access.[1] Urgent and emergency care services play a specific part in supporting patients to receive the right care, by the right person, as quickly as possible.

It makes a distinction between urgent and emergency care as follows:

- Emergency: 'Life threatening illnesses or accidents which require immediate, intensive treatment. Services that should be accessed in an emergency include ambulance (via 999) and emergency departments'
- Urgent: An illness or injury that requires urgent attention but is not a life-threatening situation. 'Urgent care services include a phone consultation through the NHS 111 Clinical Assessment Service, pharmacy advice, out-of-hours GP appointments, and/or referral to an urgent treatment centre (UTC). If unsure what service is needed, NHS 111 can help to assess and direct to the appropriate services'

The national service specification delivers an integrated 24/7 urgent care service access (referred to as IUC CAS) with the following components:

- Access to urgent care via NHS 111, either a free-to-call telephone number or online
- Triage by a health advisor
- Consultation with a clinician using a clinical decision support system (CDSS) or an agreed clinical protocol to complete the episode on the telephone where possible
- Direct booking post clinical assessment into a face-to-face service where necessary
- Electronic prescription
- Self-help information delivered to the patient

Patients are directed to the most appropriate facility based on information regarding commissioned healthcare services across England contained in the NHS Directory of Services (DoS) which includes:

- Where services are situated
- When those services are open

- The staff and skillsets they employ
- The types of clinical presentations they are commissioned to respond to
- The referral method they accept
- The patient cohort they accept
- Service capacity
  The new Ambulance Response Programme (ARP) (covered elsewhere) aims to:
- Change the way ambulance services operate in England to release efficiencies
- Provide a more clinically focused response to all 999 calls
- Improve ambulance service efficiency and stability through a new system of call handling and prioritisation
- Reduce long waits and improve the speed of response in rural areas
  The IUC CAS involves a new primary care response with the intention that:
- The vast majority of urgent care will continue to be supplied by general practice during opening hours
- General practice now offers same day and pre-bookable evening and weekend appointments
- Extended access appointments are bookable from NHS 111

Settings for Patient Care

Coordination of urgent and unscheduled care activity is essential; relevant services might include:

- Clinical advice and treatment in particular facilities (i.e. urgent treatment centres)
- Home visits (GP)
- Community nurse visits
- Palliative care teams
- Mental health assessment, help and advice
- Emergency dental services
- Social services emergency duty teams
- Pharmacy services
- Elderly care
- Dental services
  There is evidence that NHS 111 currently directs more people to accident and emergency (A&E) than need to go because the NHS Pathways algorithm by itself lacks flexibility. It is thought that if more NHS 111 callers received clinical advice, fewer people would be directed to A&E. This led to the generation of a pilot study which showed:
- A clinical advice service can reduce the number of callers being advised to attend A&E
- When NHS 111 directed patients in the North East to alternatives rather than an A&E, 82% did not require subsequent redirection to an A&E
- However, the overall effect on the proportion of callers advised to attend A&E is more modest, since only around a fifth of callers who would have been advised to attend A&E were deemed appropriate clinically to refer to a CAS. In the North East, the overall proportion of NHS 111 callers advised to attend A&E reduced from 8.0% to 6.4% as a result of this intervention (i.e. a reduction of around 20%)
- We know that many people who are advised not to go to A&E do not adhere to advice; this may be improved by:
  - Increased clinical input
  - Immediately bookable GP appointments
  - Immediately bookable UTC appointments

- NHS 111 being able to issue repeat and new prescriptions
- Targeting other behavioural factors (e.g. how advice is phrased)

Urgent Treatment Centres

The core standards of UTCs include[2]:
- GP-led, staffed by GPs, nurses and other clinicians
- Open at least 12 hours a day, every day
- Access to investigations including swabs, pregnancy tests and urine dipstick and culture, near patient blood testing, such as glucose, haemoglobin, D-dimer and electrolytes, ECG and possibly near-patient troponin
- Offers the ability to access urgent appointments within 4 hours and booked through NHS 111, ambulance services and general practice
- Offers a walk-in access option
- Equipped to diagnose and deal with many of the most common ailments people attend A&E for
- Eases the pressure on hospitals, leaving other parts of the system free to treat the most serious cases
- Offers activity that will result in decreased attendance at A&E or, in co-located services, offer the opportunity for streaming at the front door
- All UTCs considered a Type 3 A&E
- Is part of locally integrated urgent and emergency care services working in conjunction with the ambulance service, NHS 111, local GPs, hospital A&E services and other local providers
- Has protocols in place to manage critically ill and injured adults and children who arrive at UTC unexpectedly; these will usually rely on support from the ambulance service for transport to the correct facility
- Provides a full resuscitation trolley and drugs, and at least one member of staff trained in adult and paediatric resuscitation at all times
- Can issue prescriptions, including repeat prescriptions and e-prescriptions

Professional Roles in Urgent Care

The Joint National IUC CAS and NHS 111 Workforce Development Programme[3]:
- Requires personnel working over several areas including:
  - Non-clinical telephone/remote workforce
  - Clinical telephone/remote workforce
  - Mental health and wellbeing
- Comprises the following workforce:
  - Paramedics
  - Nurses (various levels)
  - Healthcare assistants
  - GPs
  - Specialised clinicians, mental health, dental health, midwifery, pharmacy and paediatrics
The NHS workforce blueprint aims to[4]:
- Raise the profile of the service
- Actively recruit new staff
- Promote IUC/NHS 111 as a career for life

Communication in Healthcare Settings

Several models exist describing communication and the optimising of relationships between clinicians, other professionals and patients.

The Relationship: Establishment, Development and Engagement (REDE) model[5] involves three phases:

- Phase 1 – establish the relationship:
  - Create a safe and supportive atmosphere
  - Build up an 'emotion bank account'
  - Convey value and respect when greeting
  - Create a climate conducive to the development of trust by demonstrating interested in the person (first) over patient (second)
  - Collaboratively set the agenda
  - 'Introduce' use of IT
  - Demonstrate empathy
- Phase 2 – develop the relationship:
  - Show genuine curiosity and interest
  - Get to know the patient as a person, understanding symptoms in a biopsychosocial context
  - Continue to deposit into the 'emotion bank account'
  - Listen reflectively
  - Elicit the patient narrative
  - Elicit the patient's perspective
- Phase 3 – engage the relationship:
  - Align with the education and treatment element of the encounter
  - Improve patient comprehension
  - Share diagnosis and information
  - Frame information in the context of the patient's perspective
  - Ask clarifying questions
  - Collaboratively develop a plan
  - Provide closure
  - Talk and communicate throughout

Consultation Models

Numerous models have been developed to describe the essential interaction between clinician and patient, with most research (and therefore description) involving doctors. The understanding of different consultation models allows for optimisation of information exchange and provides a common terminology, which is useful when training clinicians and discussing cases.

Good consultations are considered to occur when[6]:

- The patient has a single straightforward problem that is recognised and treated appropriately
- The patient has difficult or puzzling symptoms that are correctly analysed
- The clinician can add value and offer opportunistic interventions
- Decisions and clinical actions treating the patient make a difference
- Time constraints are managed well
- The patient feels better and is grateful, creating mutual satisfaction

Factors that might influence the consultation include:

- Clinician factors:
  - Tired, overworked
  - Bad/low mood

- Confidence
- Stressed (including running late)
- Patient factors:
  - Anxiety
  - Pain, fear
  - Unreasonable expectations regarding clinician / outcome
  - Multiple and complex problems
- The relationship between the clinician and patient:
  - Patient does not feel listened to
  - Feels rushed
  - Personal interaction
  - Misunderstanding/poor communication
  - Accents/language, communication barriers
- Extraneous factors:
  - Environment – noisy, hot, cold
  - Distractions – traffic, smells
  - Poor seating arrangements
  - Interruptions – signatures
  - Computer fixation
  - Technical – printer jams
  - Room layout, safety barriers (including at reception)

  Consultation models:
- Help provide a framework and shared terminology to understand and describe encounters
- Are all only partially complete
- Are likely to include five key stages:
  - Find out why the patient has come
  - Work out what's wrong
  - Explain the problem(s) to the patient
  - Develop a management plan for the patient's problem(s)
  - Use the time well and efficiently
  - …and sometimes look after yourself!
- Some are more focused on the tasks of the consultation (what needs to be achieved by the clinician)
- Others are more concerned with the process of consultation – both task and process are important and, like the yin and yang, together they make a complete whole

  Well-known and established consultation models include:
- The traditional medical interview: an example of a doctor-centred, task-focused consultation process:
  - Patient presents symptoms
  - Doctor asks questions and examines patient
  - Doctor pronounces diagnosis and/or treatment
  - Patient goes away
- The Pendleton model: another task-focused model, but more patient-centred than the traditional medical interview:
  - Find out why the patient has come, including the problem (cause, effects, history) and the patient's ideas, concerns and expectations
  - Consider other problems
  - Choose (with the patient) an appropriate action for each problem
  - Achieve a shared understanding of the problems

- Involve the patient in management and encourage them to accept appropriate responsibility
- Use time and resources appropriately
- Establish or maintain a relationship with the patient which helps to achieve the other tasks
- This model moves away from 'doctor-centredness' but is very task-focused
- The Helman folk model: a patient-centred model that suggests that any patient comes to a doctor looking for six answers, clearly expressed or not; to be effective, the clinician may need to help the patient verbalise these questions so they can be addressed:
  - What has happened?
  - Why has it happened?
  - Why to me?
  - Why now?
  - What would happen if nothing was done about it?
  - What should I do about it or whom should I consult for further help?
- Michael Balint (in 'The Doctor, His Patient and the Illness) noted that:
  - Clinicians and patients develop an emotional relationship during the consultation
  - Sometimes clinicians and patients collude about what to tackle
  - The feelings that arise in a clinician during a consultation may well be coming from the patient (counter-transference)
  - Attentive listening helps patients feel better (even if not much else changes)
  - The clinician is one of the most powerful therapeutic agents in the consultation (the doctor as drug)
  - A sick or troubled parent (usually the mother) may present their (well) child or baby as the 'symptom' (the child as the presenting complaint)
  - Some consultations extend over a period of years and both patient and doctor invest their time and attention in this process, building up a bank of resources, trust and understanding
  - The clinician may have a 'magician-like' function and be perceived (either by themselves, the patient or both) as holding all the answers up their sleeves (the 'apostolic function' of the doctor)
  - Clinicians who ask a lot of questions in the consultation get answers to their questions and no more (hence the need for open questions)
  - Clinicians must learn listening as a new skill, requiring a change in personality (asking questions only gets you answers)
- Byrne and Long discovered many doctors appeared to lack tools to deal effectively with the psychological or social aspects of the consultation, noting the following stages:
  - The doctor establishes a relationship with the patient
  - The doctor attempts to discover or actually discovers the reason for the patient's attendance
  - The doctor conducts a verbal or physical examination, or both
  - The doctor alone, the doctor and patient together, or the patient alone (in that order of probability) consider(s) the condition
  - The doctor, and occasionally the patient, details the treatment or further investigation
  - The consultation is ended, usually by the doctor
  - Byrne and Long observed:
    - Individual doctors do not have much of a repertoire of consultation skills, but tend to use the same well-worn techniques with all patients
    - The section of the consultation that comes just after the patient's initial response to the clinician's opening is one of the most significant parts of the consultation
    - Patients feel better in consultations that are more patient-centred

- Doctors who ask more open questions tend to see their patients less frequently
- Doctors often misinterpret non-verbal communication

- Roger Neighbour's 'The Inner Consultation' (one of the most important consultation models written) describes an intuitive five-stage model:
    - Connecting – developing rapport with the patient, starting in the first few moments of the consultation and continuing right through it, helps the clinician to tune in to the patient, get on the same wavelength and be empathic. Once rapport is established, the clinician explores the patient's story and gathers enough information to enable them to summarise.
    - Summarising – This stage of the consultation had not formed part of previously described models but is now well recognised as being extremely useful; helps to know enough about why the patient has come, their hopes, feelings and worries and can check this out with the patient.
    - Handing over – Clinician and patient jointly agree on a management plan and hand control back to the patient.
    - Safety-netting – A three-part safety net helps secure the consultation; there are backup plans in case the clinician is wrong and/or something unexpected happens.
    - Housekeeping – Recognises the importance of the clinician staying in good shape, dealing with any negative feelings or stress that has arisen during the consultation before the next patient arrives in the room.
- The Calgary–Cambridge approach: describes the skills needed at each stage of the consultation in order to improve communication between clinician and patient:
    - Initiating the session
    - Establishing initial rapport
    - Identifying reasons for the consultation
    - Negotiating an agenda that includes both the patient's and the clinician's needs
    - Gathering information
    - Encouraging the patient to tell their story and to explain 'why now?'
    - Using open- and closed-ended questions to explore the problem
    - Noticing both verbal and non-verbal cues
    - Finding out ideas, concerns and expectations
    - Providing structure to the consultation
    - Building the relationship
    - Developing rapport
    - Recording notes unobtrusively
    - Accepting the legitimacy of the patient's view and feelings
    - Demonstrating sensitivity, empathy and support, thinking aloud
    - Explanation and planning
    - Giving information in digestible chunks
    - Checking understanding
    - Timing explanations carefully so that, for example, reassurance is not given too early
    - Using diagrams, models and written information to help explanation
    - Closing the session
    - Summarising
    - Clarifying the agreed upon plan
- Narrative-based primary care: developed by John Launer, recognises that most patients don't come in and present a logical and coherent set of symptoms. Instead we see patients with un-sifted and unsorted problems, so there tends to be an eclectic mixture that includes:
    - Some symptoms that may go together and form a pattern

- Some that don't fit easily
- The family and social situation
- The patient's past experience of their own illnesses or those of family members
- Acknowledgement that people create or write stories in their heads in order to make sense of what has happened, and then tell these stories to other people. Like all stories, they get slightly modified in the process of 'telling'. Patients usually describe their experience in a way that slightly distorts what actually happened
- Techniques to help understand patients' stories include:
  - Circular questioning – to get away from the linear concept of cause and effect, and instead help the patient to focus on meaning, or the problem within the context of the family; for example, picking up the words that the patient has used and then using them to form open questions
  - Focusing on listening – that is not making any notes until the end of the consultation
  - Context – other than the medical context, consider the family, the workplace, faith community or other clinicians that the patient has seen
  - Creating a joint story – clinicians have contexts and stories of their own and developing a new and joint story helps emphasise the equality of the relationship between clinician and patient
  - The power balance – deliberately shifting the balance of power in the consultation so that the patient has more than usual
  - Genograms – constructing a family tree with the patient can help doctors to understand the contexts of a patient's problems much better. For example, it may reveal stories from the past that are still weaving their spells or magic in the patient's present.
- The Six 'S' model[7]:
  - Status – how we perceive people, how we behave with others and how this affects how they perceive us? In turn, this affects the course of the consultation for good or bad. The authors describe a mid-level point as being ideal – neither aloof nor arrogant, but equally not timid or apologetic
  - Story – making a connection with the patient, letting them tell their story, demonstrating that you are listening, finding out thoughts, hopes and fears (does the story have a subplot?) and taking account of cultural differences
  - Summarising – reviewing what has been said so far in a neutral and non-judgmental way – the clinician acknowledges what has been said, the patient feels listened to, there is opportunity for clarification, and mutual trust is built
  - Sharing – a change of emphasis from data gathering to problem management in a way that incorporates the patient's thoughts and hopes, as well as the doctor's views, and produces a shared plan where risk is shared as well
  - Securing – this includes safety-netting and sharing risk but also reminds us to 'secure the evidence' by making effective contemporaneous notes
  - Sanity – this section acknowledges the mental and emotional pitfalls of our work and looks at strategies to manage them

Monitoring the Delivery of Patient Care

The delivery of patient care can be monitored by National Health Service England (NHSE) and providers over a number of levels[8]:
- High-level (regulatory)
- Formal returns and 'access standards' (targets)

- Provider-based including patient satisfaction

Higher level monitoring is performed by a number of organisations who liaise between patients, the public and the NHS, with roles that include:

- Representing the views of patients and the public to the NHS
- Monitoring how well NHS bodies perform in taking account of these views
- Supporting patients who are having difficulty with NHS services; for example, in finding a service or in making a complaint

The overall structure and organisation of the NHS in England is a detailed one, involving commissioners and providers:

- The Care Quality Commission (CQC):
  - The independent regulator of all health and adult social care in England
  - Has the power to fine, prosecute or close down providers which fail to meet standards
  - Key principles include placing the views of service users at the centre of the system
  - Undertakes inspections that measure organisations in five main areas
    - Caring
    - Effectiveness
    - Responsiveness
    - Safety
    - Leadership
  - Experience shows that good and bad performance is typically related to:
    - Leadership
    - Organisational culture
    - Compassionate care
    - Safe staffing levels
    - Consistent incident reporting and learning lessons
- NHS Improvement:
  - Operates to protect and promote the interests of patients by ensuring that the whole sector works for their benefit
  - Ensures that:
    - Public sector providers are well led so that they can provide high-quality care to local communities
    - Essential NHS services continue if a provider gets into difficulty
    - The NHS payment system rewards quality and efficiency
    - Choice and competition operate in the best interests of patients
- Healthwatch England:
  - The independent consumer champion that gathers and represents the public's views on health and social care services in England
  - The national consumer champion in health and care
  - Has significant statutory powers to ensure the voice of the consumer is strengthened and heard by those who commission, deliver and regulate health and care services
  - The Health and Social Care Act formalises the relationship between Healthwatch England, the Secretary of State, NHS England, Care Quality Commission, NHS Improvement and English local authorities
- NHS Complaints Advocacy:
  - Helps patients to make a complaint about their NHS care or treatment in many areas in England
  - Free, confidential and independent of the NHS

Targets

Standards and performance targets can be useful for[9]:
- Incentivising and encouraging improvements in care and outcomes
- Providing assurance on quality and availability of care when people need it
- In some cases, the same targets can restrict the ability to innovate or result in other unintended consequences
  The current national access standards in urgent and emergency care are:
- A maximum 4-hour wait in A&E from arrival to admission, transfer or discharge
- All ambulance trusts to
  - Respond to Category 1 calls in 7 minutes on average, and respond to 90% of Category 1 calls in 15 minutes
  - Respond to Category 2 calls in 18 minutes on average, and respond to 90% of Category 2 calls in 40 minutes
  - Respond to 90% of Category 3 calls in 120 minutes
  - Respond to 90% of Category 4 calls in 180 minutes
  The NHS Access Standards Review (starting in 2018) examined the core set of NHS access standards in the context of the NHS Long Term Plan model and the latest clinical and operational evidence, in order to:
- Promote safety and outcomes
- Drive improvements in patient's experience
- Ensure the sickest and most urgent patients are given priority
- Ensure patients get the right service in the right place
  An interim report (March 2019) examined the current standards, and in particular the headline 4-hour access standard, noting:
- While it has proved useful in focusing on flow in the best hospitals and permits comparison of individual healthcare organisations and health systems, the changing nature of urgent and emergency care services means the current single standard only offers a limited insight into patient care. Specifically:
  - It does not measure total waiting times (it only reports performance during the first 4 hours and is therefore blind to the additional length of time patients spend in departments beyond this point)
  - Because it does not measure total time, departments with the same headline performance may be performing very differently in reality
  - It does not differentiate between severity of condition (it gives no insight or assurance into how departments are managing the most life-threatening illnesses)
  - It focuses on completion of treatment, whereas, for life-threatening conditions, it is the timely commencement of treatment that is crucial
  - It measures a single point in often very complex patient pathways and therefore leads to a false perception that delivery against the standard is the sole responsibility of those working within emergency departments
  - There is strong evidence that hospital processes, rather than clinical judgement, are resulting in admissions or discharge in the immediate period before a patient breaches the standard – patients are 'sucked in' as the clock approaches 4 hours
  - It is not well understood by the public who perceive that 4 hours is the time for a patient first to be seen, rather than for their treatment to be completed or to be admitted, transferred or discharged
  'Patient experience' is[10]:
- What the process of receiving care feels like for the patient, their family and caregivers
- A key element of quality, alongside providing clinical excellence and safer care

- The way that the health system delivers its care and support services – from the way the phone is answered, to the way a clinician examines them or explains what is happening – it has an impact on the experience the patient has; if safe care and clinical excellence are the 'what' of healthcare, then experience is the 'how'
- Starting with the patient, listening to their needs, and designing the experience to meet these needs is achievable and results in an environment where individual patients feel cared for and supported
  Patient and public engagement involves:
- The active participation of patients, caregivers, community representatives, community groups and the public in how services are planned, delivered and evaluated
- Broader and deeper than traditional consultation
- Involves the ongoing process of developing and sustaining constructive relationships, building strong, active partnerships and holding a meaningful dialogue with stakeholders
- Can happen at two levels:
  - Individual level – 'my say' in decisions about my own care and treatment
  - Collective level – 'my' or 'our say' in decisions about commissioning and delivery of services
- Means involving patient cohorts (patients with common conditions) in helping to get the service right for them
- About engaging the public in decisions about the commissioning, planning, design and reconfiguration of health services, either pro-actively as design partners, or reactively through consultation
- Leads to improvements in health services and is part of everyone's role in the NHS
  Patients consider the following factors important:
- Being treated as a person, not a number
- Staff who listen and spend time with patient
- Individualised treatment and no labelling
- Using language that is easy to understand
- Finding out about the latest technologies and innovations, medications
- Feeling informed, receiving information and being given options
- Efficient processes
- Knowledgeable health professionals
- Aftercare support
- Positive outcomes
- Continuity of care
- Good relationships and positive attitudes among staff
- The value of support services
  The NHS National Quality Board Patient Experience Framework outlines those elements that are critical if patients are to have a positive experience of NHS Services:
- Respect of patient-centred values, preferences, and expressed needs, including: cultural issues, the dignity, privacy and independence of patients and service users; an awareness of quality-of-life issues; and shared decision-making
- Coordination and integration of care across the health and social care system
- Information, communication and education – on clinical status, progress, prognosis and processes of care in order to facilitate autonomy, self-care and health promotion
- Physical comfort – including pain management, help with activities of daily living, and clean and comfortable surroundings
- Emotional support and alleviation of fear and anxiety – about such issues as clinical status, prognosis and the impact of illness on patients, their families and their finances

- Welcoming the involvement of family and friends, on whom patients and service users rely, in decision-making and demonstrating awareness and accommodation of their needs as caregivers
- Transition and continuity — to do with information that will help patients care for themselves away from a clinical setting, and coordination, planning and support to ease transitions
- Access to care — with attention, for example, to time spent waiting for admission or time between admission and placement in a room in an inpatient setting, also waiting time for an appointment or visit in the outpatient, primary care or social care setting
  Multiple ways to collect patient feedback exist:
- Surveys and questionnaires — includes friends and family test (FFT)
- Patient participation groups/patient panels/service user groups
- Focus groups and one-to-one interviews — group of participants who are invited to share their thoughts, feelings, attitudes and ideas on certain subjects, with the guidance of a facilitator — deeper understanding in an identified service improvement area
- Patient stories — a powerful way of engaging staff, including senior leaders
- Patient experience trackers
  The NHS 'Friends and Family Test':
- An important feedback tool that supports the fundamental principle that people who use NHS services should have the opportunity to provide feedback
- Asks people if they would recommend the services they have used and offers a range of responses
- Invites feedback on the overall experience of using the service
- Provides a mechanism to highlight both good and poor patient experience
- Has produced the biggest source of patient opinion in the world
- Indicates that at least 9 out of 10 patients would recommend the NHS services they used to their loved ones
- Is used in NHS organisations across the country to stimulate local improvement and empower staff to carry out the sorts of changes that make a real difference to patients and their care.

Applying Principles of Equality and Diversity

Equality and diversity[11] is a term used in the United Kingdom to define and champion equality, diversity and human rights as defining values of society. It promotes equality of opportunity for all, giving every individual the chance to achieve their potential, free from prejudice and discrimination.

UK legislation requires public authorities to promote equality in everything that they do, also making sure that other organisations meet their legal duties to promote equality while also doing so themselves.

In the United Kingdom under the Equality Act 2010 there are certain legal requirements under existing legislation to promote equality in the areas of nine protected characteristics:

- Age: The Act protects people of all ages. However, different treatment because of age is not unlawful direct or indirect discrimination if it can be justified (if you can demonstrate that it is a proportionate means of meeting a legitimate aim). Age is the only protected characteristic that allows employers to justify direct discrimination.
- Disability: The Act has made it easier for a person to show that they are disabled and protected from disability discrimination. Under the Act, a person is disabled if they have a physical or mental impairment which has a substantial and long-term adverse effect on their ability to carry out normal day-to-day activities, which would include things like using a telephone, reading a book or using public transport. The Act puts a duty on the employer to make reasonable

adjustments for staff to help them overcome disadvantages resulting from an impairment (e.g. by providing assistive technologies to help visually impaired staff use computers effectively). It now includes a new protection from discrimination arising from disability; it is discrimination to treat a disabled person unfavourably because of something connected with their disability (e.g. a tendency to make spelling mistakes arising from dyslexia). This type of discrimination is unlawful where the employer or other person acting for the employer knows, or could reasonably be expected to know, that the person has a disability. This type of discrimination is only justifiable if an employer can show that it is a proportionate means of achieving a legitimate aim.

- Gender reassignment (new definition): provides protection for transsexual people. A transsexual person is someone who proposes to, starts or has completed a process to change his or her gender. The Act no longer requires a person to be under medical supervision to be protected – so a woman who decides to live as a man but does not undergo any medical procedures would be covered.
- Marriage and civil partnership: protects employees who are married or in a civil partnership against discrimination; single people are not protected.
- Pregnancy and maternity: a woman is protected against discrimination on the grounds of pregnancy and maternity during the period of her pregnancy and any statutory maternity leave to which she is entitled. During this period, pregnancy and maternity discrimination cannot be treated as sex discrimination. It is necessary to take into account an employee's period of absence due to pregnancy-related illness when making a decision about her employment. Breastfeeding is now explicitly protected and needs to be brought to the attention of the providers.
- Race: includes colour, nationality and ethnic or national origins
- Religion or belief: includes any religion and no religion. It does not include political beliefs, scientific beliefs or supporting sports teams.
- Sex: both men and women are protected under the Act
- Sexual orientation: protects bisexual, gay, heterosexual and lesbian people

The Equality Act 2010 and Health and Social Care Act 2012 impose legal duties to address health inequalities, which include the need for public authorities (like the NHS) to have due regard to the need to:

- Eliminate unlawful discrimination, harassment and victimisation and other conduct prohibited by the Act
- Advance equality of opportunity between people who share a protected characteristic and those who do not
- Foster good relations between people who share a protected characteristic and those who do not

Available data shows that there are inequalities in access, health outcomes and service experience between groups of people with different characteristics and across geographies. For example:

- The GP Patient Survey shows variation by ethnicity in patient confidence and trust in their GP, (white) British 66%, compared with Chinese 44%, Bangladeshi 52% and Pakistani 52%
- Gay and Lesbian people are 1.7 times more likely than heterosexual people to report being a regular smoker
- Gay and lesbian people are 2.5 times more likely than heterosexual people to report a long-term mental health problem
- 45% of parents and caregivers of children with a physical disability, and 49% of those with children with a mental health condition or learning disability, said that staff were definitely aware of their child's medical history. This compared with 59% of parents and caregivers whose children did not have these needs.

References

1. NHSE. *Integrated Urgent Care Service Specification.* https://www.england.nhs.uk/wp-content/uploads/2014/06/Integrated-Urgent-Care-Service-Specification.pdf. Accessed 24 May 2020.
2. NHSE (o). Urgent treatment centres – principles and standards. https://www.england.nhs.uk/publication/urgent-treatment-centres-principles-and-standards/. Accessed 24 May 2020.
3. NHSE. *Integrated Urgent Care Service Specification.* https://www.england.nhs.uk/wp-content/uploads/2014/06/Integrated-Urgent-Care-Service-Specification.pdf. Accessed 24 May 2020.
4. NHSE and Health Education England. *Integrated Urgent Care / NHS 111 Workforce Blueprint.* https://www.england.nhs.uk/wp-content/uploads/2018/03/career-of-choice.pdf. Accessed 24 May 2020.
5. Windover AK, Boissy A, Rice TW, et al. The REDE model of healthcare communication: optimizing relationship as a therapeutic agent. *J Patient Exp.* 2014;1(1):8–13. https://doi.org/10.1177/237437431400100103.
6. Breckman B. The naked consultation – a practical guide to primary care consultation skills. *Nurs Stand.* 2007;21(40):30. https://doi.org/10.7748/ns2007.06.21.40.30.b630.
7. Watson A, Gillespie D. *Status and Sanity: The Modern Guide to GP Consulting: Six S for Success.* Radcliffe Publishing Ltd.; 2013.
8. Henderson R. *Monitoring the NHS.* https://patient.info/doctor/monitoring-the-nhs. Accessed 24.05.20.
9. NHSE. Clinically-led review of NHS access standards. https://www.england.nhs.uk/clinically-led-review-nhs-access-standards/. Accessed 24 May 2020.
10. NHS Institute for Innovation and Improvement. *The Patient Experience Book: A Collection of the NHS Institute for Innovation and Improvement's Guidance and Support.* https://www.england.nhs.uk/improvement-hub/wp-content/uploads/sites/44/2017/11/Patient-Experience-Guidance-and-Support.pdf. Accessed 24 May 2020.
11. NHSE. *NHS England Response to the Specific Duties of the Equality Act: Equality Information Relating to Public Facing Functions.* https://www.england.nhs.uk/wp-content/uploads/2016/02/nhse-specific-duties-equality-act.pdf. Accessed 24 May 2020.

Clinical

Providing Urgent Medical Care

Emergency and Time-Critical Conditions

Anaphylaxis (Fig. 7.1)

Classic history	• Exposure to allergen
	• Respiratory: lip, tongue, oropharynx swelling/wheeze/shortness of breath (SOB)/tightness/hypoxia
	• Skin: flushing, itching, urticaria, angio-oedema
	• Cardiovascular system (CVS): Faint, dizzy, decreased consciousness
	• Gastro-intestinal (GI): Nausea, vomiting, diarrhoea, cramping
	• Classic allergens:
	• Vaccines
	• Latex
	• Drugs: antibiotics, heparin, neuromuscular blocking agents, iron injections, anti-inflammatory analgesics, contrast media
	• Hyposensitising agents
	• Insect bites and stings – wasp, bee
	• Blood products
	• Foods: especially peanuts, almonds, walnut, fish, milk
Classic findings	• As above, particular caution if:
	• Airway swelling
	• Hypotension
	• Increasing wheeze/SOB

Anaphylaxis – cont'd

Important differential diagnoses	• Sepsis • Angio-oedema • PE • Anxiety • Asthma • Hypoglycaemia • Seizures
Potential investigations	• Regular/continuous monitoring • ECG • Bloods including lactate
Interventions and disposal options	• Airway Breathing Circulation (ABC): special consideration airway management • Lie flat/raise legs/remove allergen • 100% O_2 • Adrenaline IM (early) • Salbutamol nebuliser • IV fluid • Chlorphenamine slow IV • Hydrocortisone slow IV • Admit/observe after initial treatment
Special considerations	• Beware progressive condition which may worsen • Onset/timings since exposure is relevant • Ingestion/IV likely to be more significant than topical

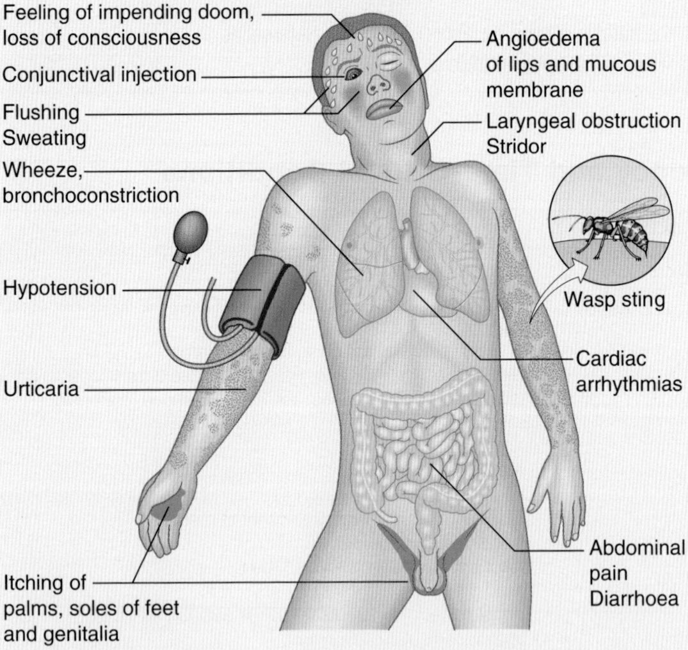

Fig. 7.1 Clinical manifestations of anaphylaxis. (From Ralston et al., 2018.)

Adult Anaphylaxis (Fig. 7.2)

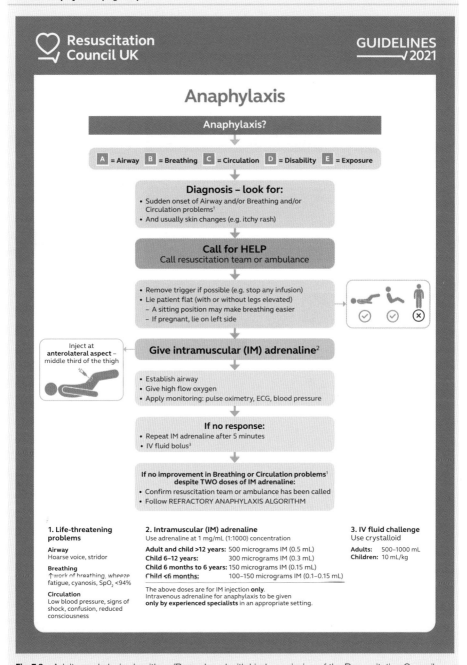

Resuscitation Council UK

GUIDELINES 2021

Anaphylaxis

Anaphylaxis?

A = Airway   B = Breathing   C = Circulation   D = Disability   E = Exposure

Diagnosis – look for:
- Sudden onset of Airway and/or Breathing and/or Circulation problems[1]
- And usually skin changes (e.g. itchy rash)

Call for HELP
Call resuscitation team or ambulance

- Remove trigger if possible (e.g. stop any infusion)
- Lie patient flat (with or without legs elevated)
  - A sitting position may make breathing easier
  - If pregnant, lie on left side

Inject at **anterolateral aspect** – middle third of the thigh

Give intramuscular (IM) adrenaline[2]

- Establish airway
- Give high flow oxygen
- Apply monitoring: pulse oximetry, ECG, blood pressure

If no response:
- Repeat IM adrenaline after 5 minutes
- IV fluid bolus[3]

If no improvement in Breathing or Circulation problems[1] despite TWO doses of IM adrenaline:
- Confirm resuscitation team or ambulance has been called
- Follow REFRACTORY ANAPHYLAXIS ALGORITHM

1. Life-threatening problems

Airway
Hoarse voice, stridor

Breathing
↑work of breathing, wheeze, fatigue, cyanosis, SpO₂ <94%

Circulation
Low blood pressure, signs of shock, confusion, reduced consciousness

2. Intramuscular (IM) adrenaline
Use adrenaline at 1 mg/mL (1:1000) concentration

Adult and child >12 years: 500 micrograms IM (0.5 mL)
Child 6–12 years: 300 micrograms IM (0.3 mL)
Child 6 months to 6 years: 150 micrograms IM (0.15 mL)
Child <6 months: 100–150 micrograms IM (0.1–0.15 mL)

The above doses are for IM injection **only**.
Intravenous adrenaline for anaphylaxis to be given **only by experienced specialists** in an appropriate setting.

3. IV fluid challenge
Use crystalloid

Adults: 500–1000 mL
Children: 10 mL/kg

Fig. 7.2 Adult anaphylaxis algorithm. (Reproduced with kind permission of the Resuscitation Council UK. The latest version can be found at: http://www.resus.org.uk.)

Cardiac Arrest (Fig. 7.3)

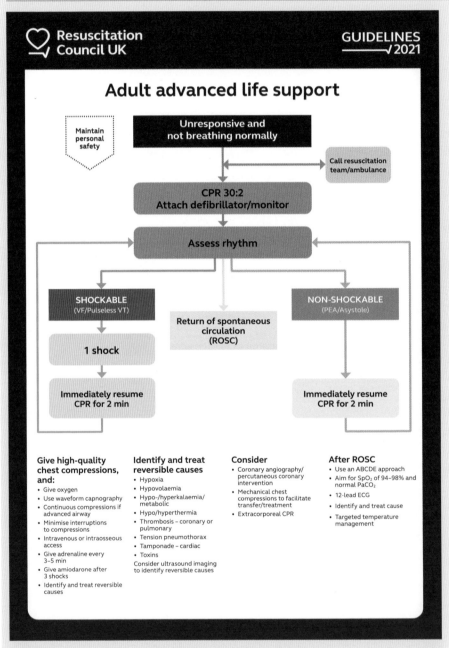

Fig. 7.3 Adult advanced life support algorithm. (Reproduced with kind permission of the Resuscitation Council UK. The latest version can be found at: http://www.resus.org.uk.)

Adult Choking (Fig. 7.4)

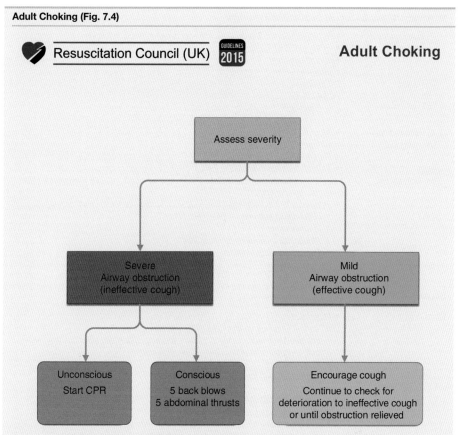

Resuscitation Council (UK)   GUIDELINES 2015   **Adult Choking**

Fig. 7.4   Adult choking algorithm. (Reproduced with kind permission of the Resuscitation Council UK. The latest version can be found at: http://www.resus.org.uk)

Meningitis/Meningococcal Septicaemia

Classic history	• Headache • Stiff neck • Photophobia • Altered consciousness • Rash • Poor feeding (child) • Seizures • Non-specific features – fever, vomiting, irritability, upper respiratory tract infection (URTI) symptoms
Classic findings	• Altered consciousness • Purpuric blanching rash/petechiae
Important differential diagnoses	• Subarachnoid haemorrhage • Migraine

Meningitis/Meningococcal Septicaemia—cont'd

UUC investigations	• Typically a clinical diagnosis with no delay for investigations
	• FBC, U&E, LFT, clotting
	• Blood cultures
	• BM
	• Glucose
	Higher level:
	  • Serology
	  • Lumbar puncture ± CT or MRI

UUC interventions and disposal	• IV or IM antibiotics immediately • IV fluids • P1 transfer and pre-alert

Special considerations	• At higher level, Indications for CT prior to lumbar puncture include:
	  • Immunocompromised state (AIDS, immunosuppressive therapy, or after transplantation)
	  • History of CNS disease (mass lesion, stroke, or focal infection)
	  • New onset seizure
	  • Papilledema
	  • Abnormal level of consciousness
	  • Focal neurologic deficit

Sepsis

Classic history	• Risk factor:
	  • Very young (<1 year) or old (>75 years)
	  • Impaired immune systems (chemotherapy, diabetes, splenectomy, sick cell, long-term steroids, immunosuppressants)
	  • Post-surgery
	  • Breach of skin (cuts burns, blisters)
	  • IV drug use
	  • Indwelling catheters/lines
	  • Pregnant, postpartum/miscarriage
	• Recent/current infection, becoming more unwell
	• Large variation in presentations so high index of suspicion is key

Classic findings and identification	• By confirming SIRS if *ANY* 2 of these:
	  • New onset confusion, altered mental state
	  • Temp >38.3c or <36c
	  • Pulse >90bpm
	  • RR >20/min
	  • Blood glucose > 7.7mmol/L (in non-diabetic)
	  • WBC >12 or <4.0
	• Thorough sepsis risk stratification if any of:
	  • SBP <90mm Hg or >40mm Hg fall from baseline
	  • MAP <65mm Hg
	  • HR >130bpm
	  • New need for supplemental O_2 to maintain saturations >90%
	  • RR >25/min
	  • AVPU=V, P or U
	  • PaO_2/FiO_2 ratio <300mm Hg or <39.9 (kPa)
	  • Lactate >2.0mmol/L
	  • Bilateral pulmonary infiltrates on CXR and new need for supplemental O_2 to maintain saturations >90%

Also refer to NICE guidelines at https://www.nice.org.uk/guidance/ng51[1] and UK Sepsis Trust at https://sepsistrust.org/professional-resources/clinical/.

Sepsis

	• Creatinine >176.8
	• INR >1.5
	• aPTT >60s
	• Platelets <100
	• Bilirubin >34.2
	• Urine output <0.5 mL/kg for 2 consecutive hours
	• Can look unwell, pale, mottled, cyanotic
Potential investigations	• FBC
	• U&E
	• CRP
	• Lactate: absolute value is related to mortality in sepsis:
	• Lactate <2: Mortality 15%
	• Lactate 2–4: Mortality 25%
	• Lactate >4: Mortality 38%
	• CXR
	• MSU dipsticks, MC&S
	• Blood cultures
Interventions and disposal options	• The 'Sepsis Six':
	• High flow oxygen
	• Blood cultures
	• IV antibiotics
	• IV fluids
	• Haemoglobin and serial lactates
	• Hourly UOP measurement
	• P1 transfer
	• Pre-alert
Special considerations	• Low threshold for consideration, do not delay potential treatment

Sepsis (Fig. 7.5)

SEPSIS SCREENING TOOL PREHOSPITAL — AGE 12+

01 START THIS CHART IF THE PATIENT LOOKS UNWELL OR NEWS2 IS 5 OR ABOVE

RISK FACTORS FOR SEPSIS INCLUDE:
- [ ] Age > 75
- [ ] Impaired immunity (e.g. diabetes, steroids, chemotherapy)
- [ ] Recent trauma / surgery / invasive procedure
- [ ] Indwelling lines / IVDU / broken skin

02 COULD THIS BE DUE TO AN INFECTION? YES

LIKELY SOURCE:
- [ ] Respiratory
- [ ] Urine
- [ ] Skin / joint / wound
- [ ] Indwelling device
- [ ] Brain
- [ ] Surgical
- [ ] Other

NO → SEPSIS UNLIKELY, CONSIDER OTHER DIAGNOSIS

03 ANY RED FLAG PRESENT? YES
- [ ] Objective evidence of new or altered mental state
- [ ] Systolic BP ≤ 90 mmHg (or drop of >40 from normal)
- [ ] Heart rate ≥ 130 per minute
- [ ] Respiratory rate ≥ 25 per minute
- [ ] Needs O$_2$ to keep SpO$_2$ ≥ 92% (88% in COPD)
- [ ] Non-blanching rash / mottled / ashen / cyanotic
- [ ] Lactate ≥ 2 mmol/l
- [ ] Recent chemotherapy
- [ ] Not passed urine in 18 hours (<0.5ml/kg/hr if catheterised)

YES → **RED FLAG SEPSIS START PH BUNDLE**

04 ANY AMBER FLAG PRESENT? NO

IF UNDER 17 & IMMUNITY IMPAIRED TREAT AS RED FLAG SEPSIS
- [ ] Relatives concerned about mental status
- [ ] Acute deterioration in functional ability
- [ ] Immunosuppressed
- [ ] Trauma / surgery / procedure in last 8 weeks
- [ ] Respiratory rate 21-24
- [ ] Systolic BP 91-100 mmHg
- [ ] Heart rate 91-130 or new dysrhythmia
- [ ] Temperature <36°C
- [ ] Clinical signs of wound infection

YES → **FURTHER INFORMATION AND REVIEW REQUIRED:**
- TRANSFER TO DESIGNATED DESTINATION
- COMMUNICATE POTENTIAL OF SEPSIS AT HANDOVER

NO AMBER FLAGS OR UNLIKELY SEPSIS: ROUTINE CARE - CONSIDER OTHER DIAGNOSIS - SAFETY-NET & SIGNPOST AS PER LOCAL GUIDANCE

PREHOSPITAL SEPSIS BUNDLE*:

RESUSCITATION:
Oxygen to maintain saturations of >94% (88% in COPD)
Measure lactate if available
250ml boluses of Sodium Chloride: max 250mls if normotensive, max 2000ml if hypotensive OR lactate >2 mmol/l

COMMUNICATION:
Pre-alert receiving hospital.
Divert to ED (or other agreed destination)
Handover presence of Red Flag Sepsis

*NICE recommends rapid transfer to hospital is the priority rather than a prehospital bundle

THE UK SEPSIS TRUST
UKST 2019 3.2 PAGE 1 OF 1
UKST, REGISTERED CHARITY 1158843

Fig. 7.5 Example of a sepsis screening and action tool. (Reproduced with permission of UK Sepsis Trust 2020, available online at https://sepsistrust.org/wp-content/uploads/2019/12/Sepsis-Prehospital-12-231219.pdf.)

Status Epilepticus

Classic history	• Continuous generalised seizure lasting >30 min, may include tongue biting, incontinence
	• Stimulus: alcohol/ drug use and withdrawal, hypoglycaemia, strobe lights, arrhythmia, head injury, subarachnoid, CVA/TIA, infection, meningitis, metabolic change
	• Complications: hypoglycaemia, pulmonary hypertension, pulmonary oedema, increased intra-cranial pressure
Important differential diagnoses	• Pregnancy-related fits (pre-eclampsia)
UUC investigations (post seizure)	• BM
	• FBC
	• U&E
	• Glucose
	• ECG
	• CXR
	• Blood cultures (if pyrexia)
	• Pregnancy test
	• Higher level:
	• Calcium
	• Magnesium
	• CT/MRI/LP once stabilised
UUC interventions and disposal	• ABC
	• Oxygen
	• IV access
	• Buccal midazolam/IV lorazepam or diazepam/rectal diazepam
	• P1 transfer with pre-alert

Unconsciousness

Important differential diagnosis	• Neurological: CVA, subarachnoid, convulsions, epilepsy Wernicke encephalopathy
	• Drugs and alcohol: intoxication, overdose
	• Head injury
	• Infection: meningitis, encephalitis, malaria, sepsis
	• Metabolic: hypoglycaemia, T2 respiratory failure, hepatorenal failure, DKA
	• Cardiac: arrhythmia, failure, arrest
	• Hypovolaemic shock
	• Anaphylaxis
	• Psychogenic
History and characteristics	• Circumstances: when last seen, how found, patterns of activity
	• Situation: trauma, drugs
	• PMHx: drugs (prescribed and recreational)
Examination considerations	• Full neurological
	• Fundoscopy
	• Respiratory depression
	• Brady or tachycardia
	• Skin: pallor, cyanosis, jaundice, rashes, injection sites, trauma
	• Temperature

Unconsciousness – cont'd

UUC investigations	• Full screen
	• BM, glucose
	• FBC
	• U&E
	• LFT
	• Clotting
	• ECG
	• CXR
	• CRP
	• Lactate
Special considerations	• ABC
	• Rapid transfer/admission
	• Higher level investigations:
	• ABG
	• CT
	• Drug levels
	• Lumbar puncture

Dealing With Symptoms

2WW – Childhood Cancers – NICE Guidelines[2]

- Neuroblastoma:
  - Consider very urgent referral (for an appointment within 48h) for specialist assessment for neuroblastoma in children with a palpable abdominal mass or unexplained enlarged abdominal organ
- Retinoblastoma:
  - Consider an urgent referral (for an appointment within 2 weeks) for ophthalmological assessment for retinoblastoma in children with an absent red reflex
- Wilms tumour:
  - Consider very urgent referral (for an appointment within 48h) for specialist assessment for Wilms' tumour in children with any of the following:
    - A palpable abdominal mass
    - An unexplained enlarged abdominal organ
    - Unexplained visible haematuria

2WW – Non-Site-Specific Symptoms – NICE Guidelines[3]

- Symptoms of concern in children or young adults:
  - Take into account the insight and knowledge of parents and carers when considering making a referral for suspected cancer in a child or young person. Consider referral for children if their parent or carer has persistent concern or anxiety about the child's symptoms, even if the symptoms are most likely to have a benign cause
- Symptoms of concern in adults:
  - For people with unexplained weight loss, which is a symptom of several cancers including colorectal, gastro-oesophageal, lung, prostate, pancreatic and urological cancer:
    - Carry out an assessment for additional symptoms, signs or findings that may help to clarify which cancer is most likely and
    - Offer urgent investigation or a 2WW referral
  - For people with unexplained appetite loss, which is a symptom of several cancers including lung, oesophageal, stomach, colorectal, pancreatic, bladder and renal cancer:
    - Carry out an assessment for additional symptoms, signs or findings that may help to clarify which cancer is most likely and
    - Offer urgent investigation or a suspected cancer pathway referral (for an appointment within 2 weeks)

2WW – Non-Site-Specific Symptoms – NICE Guidelines[3]

- For people with deep vein thrombosis, which is associated with several cancers including urogenital, breast, colorectal and lung cancer:
  - Carry out an assessment for additional symptoms, signs or findings that may help to clarify which cancer is most likely and
  - Consider urgent investigation or a suspected cancer pathway referral (for an appointment within 2 weeks)

Acute Abdominal Pain

Important differential diagnoses	• Surgical:
	  • Appendicitis
	  • Cholecystitis
	  • Pancreatitis
	  • Peptic ulcer, perforation
	  • Ruptured AAA
	  • Mesenteric infarction
	  • Diverticulitis
	  • Lage bowel perforation
	  • Intestinal obstruction
	  • Renal calculi
	  • Urinary retention
	  • Testicular torsion
	  • Intussusception
	  • Neoplasm
	• Gynaecological
	  • Ectopic pregnancy
	  • Pelvic inflammatory disease
	  • Ovarian cyst including rupture and torsion
	  • Endometriosis
	• Medical:
	  • MI
	  • Pneumonia
	  • GORD
	  • Diverticulitis
	  • Pulmonary embolus
	  • Aortic dissection
	  • Hepatitis
	  • DKA
	  • Urinary tract infection
	  • Pyelonephritis
	  • Herpes zoster
	  • Irritable bowel syndrome
	  • Inflammatory bowel disease
	  • Gastroenteritis
	• In children also consider:
	  • Mesenteric adenitis
	  • Constipation
	  • Lower lobe pneumonia
	  • Intussusception
	  • Volvulus
	  • Diabetes
	  • Henoch-Schoenlein purpura
	  • Hepatitis
	  • Colic
	  • Otitis media
	  • Non-organic

Acute Abdominal Pain – cont'd

History and characteristics	• Pain: site, radiation, timings, characteristics, precipitating and relieving factors • Vomiting: content • Bloating, distension • Change bowel habit, bleeding, mucus • Urinary, gynaecological symptoms • General: appetite, weight loss
UUC investigations	• BM • Urinalysis • Pregnancy test • FBC • U&E • LFT • Amylase • GGT • CRP • Lactate • ECG (ACS) • CXR (basal pneumonia) • AXR (if thinking obstruction, perforation, ureteric calculi)

Special considerations	• Higher level investigations:
	  • USS
	  • CT
	• If unwell/shock:
	  • ABC
	  • Oxygen
	  • IV fluids
	• Analgesia (IV morphine)
	• Antiemetic

Chest Pain

Important differential diagnoses	• Common:
	  • MSK (costochondritis/Tietze's)
	  • ACS
	  • GORD
	  • Oesophageal rupture
	  • Pneumonia
	  • Pleurisy
	  • PE
	  • Pneumothorax
	• Less common:
	  • Cholecystitis
	  • Aortic dissection
	  • Pancreatitis
	  • Neoplasm (including bony origin)
	  • Hypertrophic obstructive cardiomyopathy (HOCM)
	  • Myocarditis
	  • Biliary colic

Chest Pain

History – characteristics	• Site • Severity • Time – onset and duration • Character • Radiation • Precipitating/relieving factors • Previous similar pain • Associated – SOB, nausea, pallor, sweating, cough, dizziness, haemoptysis, GI
Examination considerations	• Full CVS/RS review • MSK (tenderness, effect of movement)
Potential investigations	• ECG • CXR • Cardiac enzymes including troponin • D-dimer
Special considerations	• Risk factors for ACS: • Age, male, smoking, BMI, diabetes, family history ischaemic heart disease, elevated cholesterol/triglycerides

Collapse/Syncope

Important differential diagnoses	• Causes of syncope:
	  • Neurological:
	    • Vasovagal attack
	    • Situational syncope
	    • Carotid-sinus syncope
	  • Psychiatric disorder:
	    • Principally panic/anxiety disorder
	  • Drug-induced
	  • Neurological disease
	  • Cardiac and vascular syncope:
	    • Structural heart disease
	    • Postural/orthostatic
	    • Arrhythmia
	• Other differential diagnoses:
	  • Mechanical trip/fall
	  • All causes of shock including GI bleed, ruptured ectopic, ruptured aortic aneurysm
	  • PE
	  • Sepsis

History and characteristics	• General history:
	  • Situation: trips/falls, relationship to events/movements, seizures, pre- and post-collapse symptoms
	  • Preceding symptoms: nausea, dizziness, yawning, darkening vision, altered hearing
	  • Confusion or weakness
	  • Tongue biting
	  • Incontinence
	  • Previous episodes
	  • Family history of sudden death aged <40 years

Collapse/Syncope – cont'd

	• More likely vasovagal if: • Obvious precipitant (warm room, triggers such as sight of blood) • Prodrome (light-headed) • Position (prolonged standing) • Post event nausea, vomiting or fatigue
Examination considerations	• Full neurological • Fundoscopy • Respiratory depression • Brady or tachycardia • Signs of tongue biting or trauma • CVS: murmurs and arrhythmias • Sitting/standing BP • Skin: pallor, cyanosis, jaundice, rashes, injection sites, trauma • Temperature • Digital rectal examination (gastro bleed)
UUC investigations	• BM, glucose • FBC, U&E, clotting • ECG • CXR
Special considerations	• Consider admission/immediate cardiology review if: • ECG abnormality • New heart failure • LOC on exertion • Family history sudden cardiac death <40 years or inherited cardiac condition • Age >65 with no prodrome • New heart murmur • Specialist neurological referral if new seizure likely • Possibly relevant higher-level investigations: • ABG • CT • Drug levels • Lumbar puncture • Tilt table • Echo • 24 hr ECG and BP • Exercise tolerance test

Haemoptysis

Important differential diagnoses	• CVS: • Pulmonary embolism • Pulmonary oedema • Respiratory • Neoplasm • Infection (including tuberculosis) • Bronchiectasis

Haemoptysis

	• Coagulation disorder
	• ENT
	  • Nosebleeds and related
	• Trauma
	• Other:
	  • Mitral stenosis
	  • Wegener granulomatosis

History and characteristics	• Associated features (excess coughing) • Colour (bright red vs dark brown) • Nature (granules) • Amount (thimble, egg cup, etc.) • Blood loss elsewhere including bruising • Smoking • Weight loss • Dysphagia • Dysphonia
Examination considerations	• Cardiovascular status – pallor, shock • Respiratory status – stridor, rate, pattern, percussion and auscultation findings • General appearance – skin including bruising and rashes, pyrexia, clubbing, cachexia, nodes

Potential investigations	• FBC, coagulation, U&Es, LFTs
	• ABG
	• CXR
	• ECG
	• Urinalysis
	• Sputum MC&S
	• Higher level:
	  • Ventilation/perfusion scan (PE)
	  • Bronchoscopy
	  • CT

Special considerations	• NICE lung cancer guidelines[4]:
	  • 2WW referral if:
	    • CXR suggests lung cancer, or
	    • Age ≥40 with unexplained haemoptysis
	  • Offer urgent CXR for people age ≥40 with 2 or more (if have never smoked), or 1 (if have ever smoked) of unexplained symptoms from:
	    • Cough
	    • Fatigue
	    • Shortness of breath
	    • Chest pain
	    • Weight loss
	    • Appetite loss
	  • 'Unexplained' is defined as 'symptoms or signs that have not led to a diagnosis being made by the healthcare professional in primary care after initial assessment (including history, examination and any primary care investigations)'
	  • Consider an urgent CXR (within 2 weeks) if age ≥40 and any of:
	    • Persistent or recurrent chest infection
	    • Finger clubbing
	    • Supraclavicular lymphadenopathy or persistent cervical lymphadenopathy
	    • Chest signs consistent with lung cancer
	    • Thrombocytosis

Hyperventilation

Important differential diagnoses	• Respiratory
	  • Infection
	  • Asthma
	  • COPD
	  • Pleural effusion
	  • Haemothorax
	  • Pneumothorax
	  • Interstitial lung disease
	• Cardiac
	  • Pulmonary oedema
	  • ACS
	  • PE
	  • Arrythmia including fast AF
	• Trauma
	  • Aspiration
	  • Foreign body
	  • Flail chest
	  • Pneumothorax
	  • Haemothorax
	• Systemic/other
	  • Pyrexia
	  • Anaemia
	  • Hypovolaemia
	  • Anxiety/stress/'hyperventilation'
	  • Diabetic keto-acidosis (DKA)
	  • Hyperthyroidism

Potential investigations	• FBC • CXR • SpO_2 • ABG

Breast

2WW – Breast – NICE Guidelines[5]

- 2WW referral for breast cancer if:
  - Aged 30 and over and have an unexplained breast lump with or without pain, or
  - Aged 50 and over with any of the following symptoms in one nipple only:
    - Discharge
    - Retraction
    - Other changes of concern
- Consider a 2WW referral for breast cancer in people:
  - With skin changes that suggest breast cancer, or
  - Aged 30 and over with an unexplained lump in the axilla
- Consider non-urgent referral in people aged under 30 with an unexplained breast lump with or without pain
- Consider beast cancer in males

Breast Lump

Classic history	• Need to assess:
	  • Age
	  • Menopausal status (pre/peri/post)
	  • Timing (cycle)
	  • Lump characteristics – discrete or diffuse, hard, or soft, firm or fluctuant, tender or non-tender
	  • Other factors – breast feeding, trauma, skin changes
	  • Previous history
	  • Family history of breast disorders
	  • Drug history
	  • Weight changes

Classic findings	• Need for chaperone • Examine breasts, skin, axillae

Important differential diagnoses	• Common painful:
	  • Mastitis
	  • Abscess
	  • Fibro-adenosis
	  • Carcinoma
	  • Tietze's/MSK
	• Common painless:
	  • Carcinoma
	  • Fibrocystic
	  • Fibroadenoma
	  • Galactocele
	  • Fat necrosis
	  • Chest wall including lipoma
	  • Gynaecomastia

Potential investigations	• Higher level:
	  • Mammogram
	  • Ultrasound scan
	  • (Guided) biopsy
	  • MRI

Mastitis

Classic history	• Tender breast area • Fever • Malaise, flu-like illness including headache, fevers and chills, myalgia
Classic findings	• Red, swollen, tender breast area • Pyrexia
Potential investigations	• Breast milk MC&S or skin swab if resistant to treatment
Interventions and disposal options	• Advice: continue breast feeding (ok for baby), consider emptying breast • Paracetamol or ibuprofen • If no improvement after 12–24 h – start antibiotics (typically flucloxacillin) • Consider abscess formation

Cardiology

Angina

Classic history	• Dull, tight or heavy chest discomfort precipitated by exertion, cold, 'stress' etc. • Radiation to jaw, arms, neck or back • Relieved by rest, GTN

Important differential diagnoses	• Cardiovascular:
	  • ACS
	  • Aortic dissection
	  • PE
	  • Aortic stenosis
	  • HOCM
	• GI:
	  • Oesophagitis
	  • GORD
	  • Biliary colic
	  • Gastritis
	  • Pancreatitis
	• MSK:
	  • Muscle strain
	  • Tietze syndrome
	• Other:
	  • Anxiety
	  • Hyperventilation

Potential investigations	• ECG (ST depression or inversion which resolves on recovery)
	• Troponin
	• FBC (anaemia)
	• CXR
	• Higher level:
	  • Exercise tolerance test
	  • CT angiography
	  • Invasive angiography

Interventions and disposal options	• Managing acute angina attack:
	  • GTN spray
	  • Repeat dose once after 5 min if pain not gone
	  • 999 P1 transfer if pain remains 5 min after second dose
	• Those with angina/suspected angina need to see their GP for referral to cardiologist if:
	  • New onset of chest pain suspected to be ischaemic of origin
	  • Exacerbation of stable angina
	  • Recurrence of old (resolved) angina
	  • Previous history of myocardial infarction, coronary artery bypass graft, or percutaneous transluminal coronary angioplasty and development of angina
	  • Evidence of previous MI or other abnormality in the initial ECG
	  • New atrial fibrillation
	  • Cardiac failure and angina
	  • Ejection systolic murmur suggesting aortic stenosis
	  • Treatment failure despite maximum therapeutic doses of two drugs
	  • Atypical symptoms, concern re diagnosis uncertainty
	  • Multiple risk factors or strong family history
	  • Significant comorbid disease, e.g. diabetes

Special considerations	• Normal ECG, baseline cardiac markers and examination does not necessarily exclude MI

Acute Coronary Syndromes – Unstable Angina/ Non ST-elevation myocardial infarction (NSTEMI)

Classic history	• Worsening angina/crescendo angina
	• Angina at rest
	• Increasing frequency, severity of pain
Classic findings	• May look well
	• Diaphoresis through to collapse
Important differential diagnosis	• Cardiovascular:
	• Angina
	• Aortic dissection
	• PE
	• Aortic stenosis
	• HOCM
	• GI:
	• Oesophagitis
	• GORD
	• Biliary colic
	• Gastritis
	• Pancreatitis
	• MSK:
	• Muscle strain
	• Tietze syndrome
	• Other:
	• Anxiety
	• Hyperventilation
Potential investigations	• ECG (no ST elevation by definition)
Interventions and disposal options	• Continuous cardiac monitoring
	• Oxygen (if SpO_2 <94%)
	• IV morphine
	• IV antiemetic
	• If diagnosis not confirmed (i.e. chest pain only) then just aspirin 300 mg. If diagnosis confirmed then dual platelet as below
	• Aspirin 300 mg plus Ticagrelor (consider bleeding diathesis), or
	• Aspirin 300 mg plus clopidogrel 300 mg (consider 600 mg particularly when PCI will be used) - consider bleeding diathesis
	• S/L GTN: 1–2 sprays every 5 min if required, max 3 doses in 15 min
	• P1 transfer: PCI/Chest Pain Assessment Unit
Special considerations	• Difficult to distinguish unstable angina from NSTEMI
	• The TIMI Risk Score predictor identifies 7 important prognosis factors of death and ischaemic events:
	• 65 years or older
	• At least 3 risk factors for coronary artery disease
	• Prior coronary stenosis of 50% or more
	• ST-segment deviation on electrocardiogram at presentation
	• At least 2 anginal events in prior 24 h
	• Use of aspirin in prior 7 days
	• Elevated serum cardiac markers[6]
	• 'Variant' (Prinzmetal) angina – angina associated with ST elevation as result of coronary artery vasospasm
	• Consider drug (i.e. cocaine)-induced which requires separate algorithm

Acute Coronary Syndromes – ST-elevation myocardial infarction (STEMI)

Classic history	• Sudden onset 'cardiac' chest pain: central, crushing
	• Radiation: jaw, neck, left arm
	• Diaphoresis and related: nausea, clamminess, sweating, SOB
	• High risk factors: smoking, hypertension, age, male, family hx IHD, hyperlipidaemia, diabetes

Acute Coronary Syndromes – ST-elevation myocardial infarction (STEMI) – cont'd

Classic findings	• Pale, sweaty
	• 'Impending doom'
	• New murmurs
	• New cardiac failure
Relevant anatomy	• Consider check peripheral pulses (aortic dissection)
Important differential diagnoses	• Cardiovascular:
	• ACS
	• Aortic dissection
	• PE
	• Aortic stenosis
	• HOCM
	• GI:
	• Oesophagitis
	• GORD
	• Biliary colic
	• Gastritis
	• Pancreatitis
	• MSK:
	• Muscle strain
	• Tietze syndrome
	• Other:
	• Anxiety
	• Hyperventilation
Potential investigations	• (Serial) ECG: changes as determined by location and phase of infarct
	• Cardiac markers (including troponin), U&E, glucose, FBC, lipids, amylase (pancreatitis)
	• Diagnosis involves at least 2 from history/ECG/cardiac marker changes
Interventions and disposal options	• Continuous cardiac monitoring
	• Oxygen (if SpO_2 <94%)
	• IV morphine
	• IV antiemetic
	• If diagnosis not confirmed (i.e. chest pain only) then just aspirin 300 mg. If diagnosis confirmed then dual platelet as below
	• Aspirin 300 mg plus ticagrelor 180 mg (consider bleeding diathesis), or
	• Aspirin 300 mg plus clopidogrel 300 mg (consider 600 mg particularly when PCI will be used) - consider bleeding diathesis
	• S/L GTN: 1–2 sprays every 5 min if required, max 3 doses in 15 min
	• P1 transfer: PCI/Chest Pain Assessment Unit
Special considerations	• Be prepared for arrythmias, cardiac arrest
	• Some areas/countries would initiate thrombolysis if PCI delayed (>90 min)

Acute Coronary Syndromes – ST-elevation myocardial infarction (STEMI) (Figs 7.6 and 7.7)

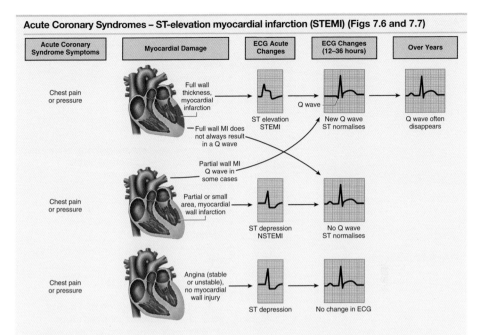

Fig. 7.6 Acute coronary syndrome: ECG changes over time. (From Urden, Stacy & Lough, 2020.)

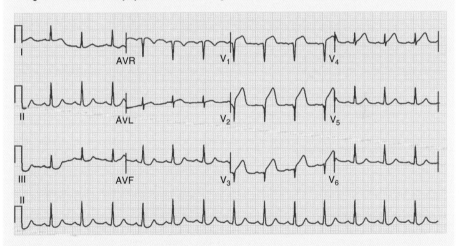

Fig. 7.7 Acute anteroseptal myocardial infarction. Note: ST segment elevation and pathological Q waves in leads V1–V3. Ischaemic changes with ST segment depression are also seen in the inferior leads (II, III and AVF). (From Feather, Randall & Waterhouse, 2021.)

Aortic Dissection

Classic history	• Sudden onset severe 'tearing' anterior or posterior chest pain • Potential radiation • Sweat, pallor • Syncope • Neurological deficit
Classic findings	• Distressed • Collapsed • Aortic regurgitation • Diaphoresis (pale, sweaty, clammy), tachycardia • Asymmetric/absent peripheral pulses • Hypertension or hypotension • Visceral/limb ischaemia
Important differential diagnoses	• ACS • PE • Pneumothorax • Renal colic • CVA (focal neurology)

Potential investigations	• U&E
	• Glucose
	• FBC
	• ECG
	• CXR (widened mediating, 'double knuckle' aorta, pleural effusion, right-sided trace deviation, separation of calcified aorta wall)
	• D-Dimer (also elevated, non-specific)
	• Higher level:
	  • CT
	  • Echo
	  • MRI

Interventions and disposal options	• Oxygen • Large bore cannula • IV morphine and antiemetic • P1 transfer – cardiothoracic

Brady and Tachy-Arrythmias (Figs 7.8 and 7.9)

Classic history	• Immediate or delayed consequence of ACS event • Palpitations, dizziness, chest pain, SOB • Features of shock
Important differential diagnoses	• Other causes of tachycardia including pain, anxiety
Potential investigations	• ECG/cardiac monitoring
Interventions and disposal options	• ABC/ILS/ALS • Oxygen • Cannula • Observe/treat features of shock (see algorithms) • P1 transfer

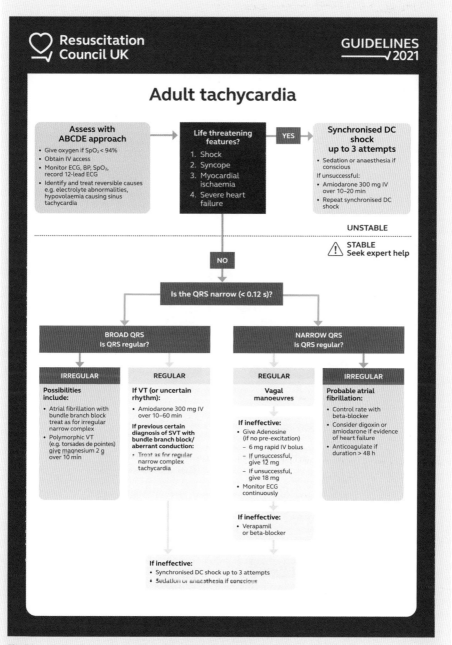

Fig. 7.8 Adult tachycardia algorithm. (Reproduced with the permission of the Resuscitation Council UK. The latest version can be found at: http://www.resus.org.uk.)

Brady and Tachy-Arrythmias

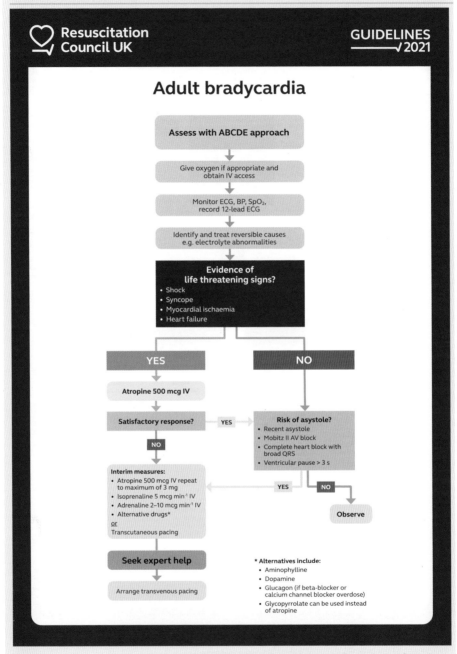

Fig. 7.9 Adult bradycardia algorithm. (Reproduced with kind permission of the Resuscitation Council UK. The latest version can be found at: http://www.resus.org.uk.)

Brady and Tachy-Arrythmias (Figs 7.8 and 7.9)

Special considerations	• Consider vagal stimulation/adenosine for stable narrow complex tachycardia
	• Driving group 1:
	  • Stop if arrhythmia did or could cause incapacity
	  • Refer to current DVLA guidelines[7]

Electrical Injury

History and characteristics	• Source of shock (current, voltage, alternating or direct current)
	• Duration of contact
	• Severity depends upon:
	  • Severity of shock dependant on intensity of current
	  • Severity of burn dependant on energy delivered (joules)
	  • Duration of contact
	  • Path taken through body
	  • Voltage of current
	  • Alternating or direct current

Examination considerations	• Assess for burns at entry and exit site
Potential investigations	• ECG

Special considerations	• Heart:
	  • Arrhythmias can be delayed for up to 12 h
	• Renal:
	  • Delayed renal failure
	• MSK:
	  • Compartment syndrome, rhabdomyolysis
	• Low concerns (if low voltage, no LOC/cardiac arrest/arrythmia): Discharge home if ECG normal
	• High voltage: admit for observation

Left Ventricular Failure/Pulmonary Oedema

Classic history	• Significant shortness of breath, often with associated distress • Fatigue • Frothy pink sputum • Wheeze
Classic findings	• Looks unwell, pale, sweaty • Fine inspiratory crepitations • Tachypnoea • Tachycardia • Cyanosis • Pink frothy sputum • Gallup rhythm • Wheeze
Important differential diagnoses	• ACS • PE • Spontaneous pneumothorax

Left Ventricular Failure/Pulmonary Oedema – cont'd

Potential investigations	• Cardiac monitor
	• FBC, U&E
	• ECG (arrythmias, LAD, LVH, LBBB, ACS)
	• CXR (pleural effusions, 'Kerley' lines, 'bat's wing' hilar shadows, upper lobe)
	• ABG
	• Higher level:
	  • BNP
	  • Echo
	  • TFT
	  • MUGA scan

Interventions and disposal options	• ABC
	• Sit patient up
	• High flow oxygen if saturation < 95%
	• Intravenous diuretic: 20–40 mg frusemide
	• Intravenous opiate analgesia: 5 mg diamorphine over 5 min (with caution)
	• GTN S/L if pain present
	• P1 transfer
	• Pre-alert
	• Higher level:
	  • Treat arrhythmias: DC cardioversion or IV anti- arrhythmic therapy
	  • IV Digoxin
	  • Venesection
	  • Inotropes

Special considerations	• NICE directs[8]: • Refer patients with suspected heart failure and previous myocardial infarction (MI) urgently, to have transthoracic Doppler 2D echocardiography and specialist assessment within 2 weeks • Measure serum natriuretic peptides (B-type natriuretic peptide (BNP) or N-terminal pro-B-type natriuretic peptide (NTproBNP)) in patients with suspected heart failure without previous MI • Refer patients with suspected heart failure and a BNP level above 400 pg/mL (116 pmol/L) or an NTproBNP level above 2000 pg/mL (236 pmol/L) urgently, to have transthoracic Doppler 2D echocardiography and specialist assessment within 2 weeks • Refer patients with suspected heart failure and a BNP level between 100 and 400 pg/mL (29–116 pmol/L) or an NTproBNP level between 400 and 2000 pg/mL (47–236 pmol/L) to have transthoracic Doppler 2D echocardiography and specialist assessment within 6 weeks

Pericarditis

Classic history	• Chest pain – sharp, retrosternal, worse deep inspiration/change position/swallowing/exercise • Pain relieved by bending forward • Low grade fever
Classic findings	• Pericardial rub • New right ventricular failure • Pulsus paradoxus • Kussmaul sign – paradoxical rise in jugular venous pressure (JVP) on inspiration, or a failure in the appropriate fall of the JVP with inspiration

Pericarditis

Important differential diagnosis	• ACS • MSK • PE • LRTI • GORD
Potential investigations	• ECG (sinus tachycardia, AF, flutter, ectopics, ST-elevation, T wave peak then inverted) • CXR • FBC • CRP • U&E • Troponin • D-dimer
Interventions and disposal options	• Analgesia (NSAIDs – indomethacin, ibuprofen) • Admit • Higher-level treatment includes aspiration of pericardial effusion
Special considerations	• Requires echo and treatment • Potential complication of pericardial effusion includes Dressler syndrome (autoimmune pericarditis ± effusion 2–14 weeks after MI)

Uncontrolled Atrial Fibrillation

Classic history	• May be asymptomatic at onset
	• SOB
	• Dizziness
	• Palpitations
	• Features of embolic impact, i.e. TIA/CVA or failure
	• May be associated with:
	  • Hypertension
	  • Sepsis
	  • Thyrotoxicosis
	  • Valvular disease
	  • CAD
	  • LRTI
	  • PE
	  • Alcohol and caffeine intake

Classic findings	• Shortness of breath • Dizziness • Palpitations • Ankle swelling
Relevant anatomy	• Most common change is fibrosis of atria

Potential investigations	• FBC
	• U&E
	• ECG
	• CXR
	• Higher level:
	  • TFT
	  • Echocardiography

Interventions and disposal options	• Cannulate
	• Treat as necessary otherwise GP/specialist f/u for:
	  • Rate control: β-blocker, digoxin
	  • Rhythm control: Class IV, I and III drugs
	  • Prevent thromboembolism: warfarin, DOAC (GP)
	  • Cardioversion

Special considerations	• Patients with rapid AF related to shock, syncope, ischaemia or failure may need cardioversion under sedation • Paroxysmal atrial fibrillation also requires anticoagulation

Uncontrolled Hypertension

Classic history	• May be asymptomatic • Severe hypertension: features of CVA, headache, nausea, vomiting, confusion • Consider recreational drugs (cocaine, ecstasy)

Classic findings	• Severe hypertension:
	  • Retinal haemorrhage, exudate, papilledema
	  • Fits
	  • Focal neurological signs
	  • Decreased conscious level

Potential investigations	• U&E • Urinalysis • CXR • ECG

Interventions and disposal options	• Moderate hypertensives with no other concerns:
	  • Ideally avoid starting new regimen if possible
	  • Consider start of additional (new) antihypertensive, i.e. β-blocker (not if caused by cocaine/amphetamine), calcium channel blocker
	  • Follow-up by GP
	• NICE suggests[9]:
	  • If blood pressure ≥ 180/120 mm Hg but no symptoms or signs, then carry out investigations for target organ damage as soon as possible, f/u with GP
	  • If target organ damage is identified, consider starting antihypertensive drug treatment immediately, without waiting for the results of ABPM or HBPM
	  • If no target organ damage is identified, repeat clinic blood pressure measurement within 7 days
	  • Refer for (same day) specialist assessment if BP ≥ 180/120 mm Hg with:
	    • Signs of retinal haemorrhage or papilledema (accelerated hypertension) or
	    • Life-threatening symptoms such as new onset confusion, chest pain, signs of heart failure, or acute kidney injury
	    • And anyway if suspected phaeochromocytoma (e.g. labile or postural hypotension, headache, palpitations, pallor, abdominal pain or diaphoresis)

Special considerations	• In pregnancy: consider pre-eclampsia

Dental

Acute Dental and Gum Infection

Classic history	• Toothache • Spontaneous pus drainage
Classic findings	• Gum erythema, swelling • Possible lymph node involvement, pyrexia

Acute Dental and Gum Infection (Figs 7.10 and 7.11)

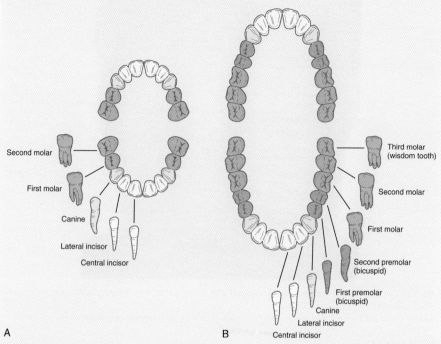

Fig. 7.10   Deciduous (A) and permanent (B) teeth; specific tooth damage should be captured in medical records. (From Zenith, 2016.)

Important differential diagnosis	• Temporo-mandibular joint (TMJ) pain • Headache • Sinusitis • Parotid pain • Trigeminal neuralgia • GCA • Abscess
Potential investigations	• FBC • Inflammatory and sepsis markers

Interventions and disposal options	• As acute treatment:
	  • Simple: oral antibiotics (amoxicillin or metronidazole or clarithromycin)
	  • Cellulitis/severe infection (including lymph node involvement, fever, malaise): amoxicillin and metronidazole (or clarithromycin and metronidazole)
	  • Analgesia
	  • Chlorhexidine rinse
	• Needs dental review

Special considerations	• Management is dental, not medical • Considerations include position of indemnity provider; they may not be happy with provision of dental care by non-dentally qualified clinicians • May be reasonable to start antibiotics and analgesia if patient is unwell and dental review would be delayed but this is not optimum treatment (dental surgical intervention is); must emphasise need for dental review • Consider whether advanced presentation may require admission

Acute Dental and Gum Infection—cont'd

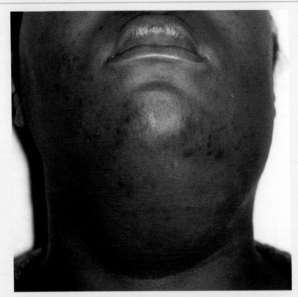

Fig. 7.11 Wider swelling and cellulitis associated with a dental infection requiring admission for intravenous antibiotics. (From Flynn, 2000.)

Dermatology

2WW – Skin – NICE Guidelines[10]

- Melanoma:
- 2WW referral for melanoma if patient has a suspicious pigmented skin lesion with a weighted 7-point checklist score of 3 or more as follows:
  - Major features of the lesions (scoring 2 points each):
    - Change in size
    - Irregular shape
    - Irregular colour
  - Minor features of the lesions (scoring 1 point each):
  - Largest diameter 7 mm or more
  - Inflammation
  - Oozing
  - Change in sensation
- 2WW referral for melanoma if dermoscopy suggests melanoma
- 2WW referral for melanoma in patients with a pigmented or non-pigmented skin lesion that suggests nodular melanoma
- Squamous cell carcinoma:
  - Consider a 2WW referral for lesions that 'raise the suspicion' of squamous cell carcinoma
- Basal cell carcinoma:
  - Consider routine referral for people if they have a skin lesion that raises the suspicion of a basal cell carcinoma (typical features of BCC include: an ulcer with a raised rolled edge; prominent fine blood vessels around a lesion; or a nodule on the skin (particularly pearly or waxy nodules)
  - Only consider 2WW referral for patients with a skin lesion that raises the suspicion of a basal cell carcinoma if there is particular concern that a delay may have a significant impact, because of factors such as lesion site or size

A Systematic Way to Describe Skin Lesions

Primary morphology	• Macule – flat lesion less than 1 cm, without elevation or depression • Patch – flat lesion greater than 1 cm, without elevation or depression • Plaque – flat, elevated lesion, usually greater than 1 cm • Papule – elevated, solid lesion less than 1 cm • Nodule – elevated, solid lesion greater than 1 cm • Vesicle – elevated, fluid-filled lesion, usually less than 1 cm • Pustule – elevated, pus-filled lesion, usually less than 1 cm • Bulla – elevated, fluid-filled lesion, usually greater than 1 cm • Wheal – elevated, irregular area of subcutaneous oedema: red, pale, pink or white
Size	• In millimetres
Demarcation	• Well-demarcated • Not well-demarcated
Colour	• White • Red • Purple • Brown • Yellow • Black • Blue
Secondary morphology	• Crusting • Ulcerated • Fissure • Lichenification • Erosion • Scaling • Excoriation • Covering (i.e. material, the 'fabric sign') • Surrounding features i.e. vessel growth
Distribution	• Location • Surface (i.e. extensor) • Generalised vs localised • Specific (i.e. photo-) distribution • Similar to surrounding or unique 'ugly duckling'
Nature	• Itchy • Tender • Warm • Swelling • Slow or rapidly growing • Trend – larger or smaller

Classic Benign Skin Conditions

General

Benign skin lesions are often (not always):

• Symmetrical in shape, colour and structure
• Stable or slowly evolving
• Absent of spontaneous bleeding and itchWhere there is any doubt patients should be referred on for further assessment which may involve dermoscopy

Classic Benign Skin Conditions – cont'd

Condition	Classic Features
Lipoma (Fig. 7.12)	• Soft, rubbery, mobile lump • Typically back, neck or trunk

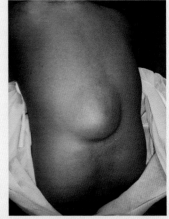

Fig. 7.12   Lipoma on back. (From Rao & Rao, 2016.)

Condition	Classic Features
Sebaceous cyst (Fig. 7.13)	• Slow growing • Round, dome-shaped lump • Yellow or white • Often with a small dark plug (punctum) • Range mm to cm

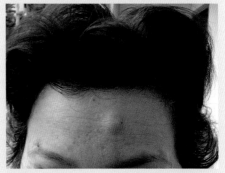

Fig. 7.13   Sebaceous cyst. (From Scully, 2010.)

Condition	Classic Features
Seborrheic keratosis (Fig. 7.14)	• Dull, waxy surface • 'Stuck on' appearance • Varied size, shape and structure • Variety of colours

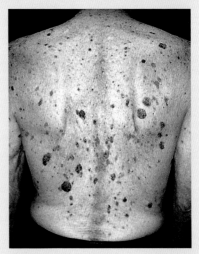

Fig. 7.14   Multiple seborrheic keratosis lesions on the trunk. (From Goldstein and Goldstein, 1997. Courtesy Department of Dermatology, Medical College of Georgia.)

Condition	Classic Features
Acne (Fig. 7.15)	• Comedones (blackheads and whiteheads) and pustules (pus-filled spots) • Classically starts during puberty and resolves by mid-twenties • Face, back, back and chest

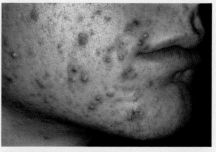

Fig. 7.15 Moderate to severe inflammatory acne. (From Dinulos, 2021.)

Condition	Classic Features
Herpes simplex (Fig. 7.16)	• Easily transferred from person • Sore or blister with tingling or tenderness • Possible local swelling • Affecting lips, genital area, hands

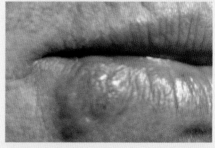

Fig. 7.16 Herpes simplex. (From Cooper & Gosnell, 2023.)

Condition	Classic Features
Folliculitis (Fig. 7.17)	• Inflamed hair follicles involving tender red spot, often with surface pustule • Superficial or deep

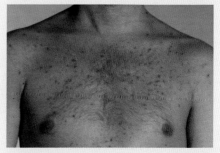

Fig. 7.17 Folliculitis on upper trunk and proximal limbs. (From Feather, Randall & Waterhouse, 2021.)

Condition	Classic Features
Impetigo (Fig. 7.18)	• Acute superficial bacterial skin infection with pustules and honey-coloured crusted erosions

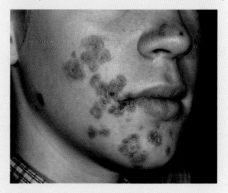

Fig. 7.18 Impetigo. (From Dinulos, 2021.)

Classic Benign Skin Conditions – cont'd

Condition	Classic Features
Atopic eczema (Fig. 7.19)	• Red, dry, itchy patches • Can weep, crust, scale and thicken • Often start at flexor surfaces elbows and knees

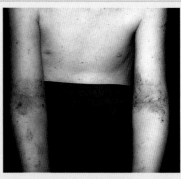

Fig. 7.19 Atopic eczema affecting elbow flexure surfaces. (With permission from the Department of Medical Illustration, St. Bartholomew's Hospital, London.)

Condition	Classic Features
Dermatitis (Fig. 7.20)	• Red, itchy, inflamed skin due to a number of underlying conditions • May be blistered and swollen • Chronic version may involve darker, thickened skin

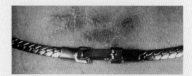

Fig. 7.20 Allergic contact dermatitis. (From Cohen, 2013.)

Condition	Classic Features
Psoriasis (Fig. 7.21)	• Symmetrically distributed, red, scaly plaques with well-defined edges • Scale typically silvery white, except in skin folds where the plaques often appear shiny and they may have a moist peeling surface • Common in scalp, elbows and knees, but any part of the skin can be involved • Itch may be severe leading to scratching and thickened leathery skin • Painful skin cracks or fissures may occur • After plaques clear may leave brown or pale marks that fade

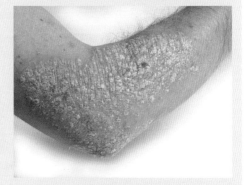

Fig. 7.21 Chronic psoriasis. (From Pizzorno & Murray, 2021.)

Condition	Classic Features
Chickenpox (Fig. 7.22)	• Itchy, red papules progressing to vesicles • Typically stomach, back and face, spreading elsewhere including inside mouth

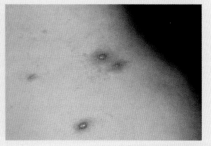

Fig. 7.22 Chickenpox. (From Paller & Mancini, 2016.)

Condition	Classic Features
Shingles (Fig. 7.23)	• Localised, blistering and painful rash • Characterised by unilateral dermatomal distribution with sharp cut-off

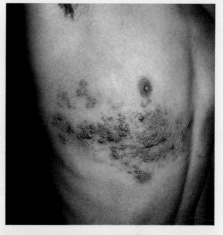

Fig. 7.23 Herpes zoster (shingles) on the anterior chest, classic dermatomal distribution. (From James, Berger & Elston, 2011.)

Condition	Classic Features
Cellulitis (Fig. 7.24)	• Localised area of red, painful, warm, swollen skin • May involve 'tracking', dimpled skin, abscess, ulceration, purpure, petechiae, lymphadenopathy • Possibly with systemic symptoms including fever, chills and shakes (rigors)

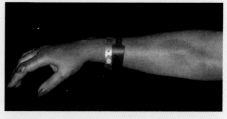

Fig. 7.24 Cellulitis that started with an injury to the index finger. (From High & Prok, 2021.)

Condition	Classic Features

Urticaria (Fig. 7.25)	• Wheals or hives:
	  • Superficial, skin-coloured or pale skin swelling lasting minutes to hours
	  • Itchy or burning sensation
	  • May be slightly raised with surrounding erythema
	  • May form rings, 'map', giant patches
	• Angioedema:
	  • Deeper swolling within the skin
	  • Red or skin-coloured
	  • Resolves within 72h
	  • May be itchy, painful or asymptomatic

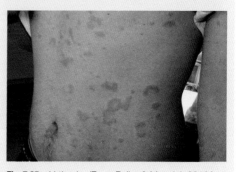

Fig. 7.25 Urticaria. (From Paller & Mancini, 2016.)

Classic Benign Skin Conditions – cont'd

Condition	Classic Features
Keloid (Fig. 7.26)	• Firm, smooth, hard growth due to spontaneous scar formation • May be uncomfortable or itchy and extend beyond original wound • May form on any part of the body, typically upper chest and shoulders

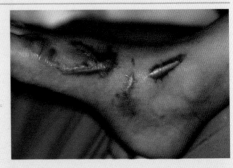

Fig. 7.26 Keloid scars. (From Dockery et al., 2012.)

Solar Lentigo (Fig. 7.27)	• Pigmented macule arising as a result of prolonged exposure to sun therefore typically occur in older population • Vary in size, typically brown/black or tan • Uniformly pigmented with sharp border

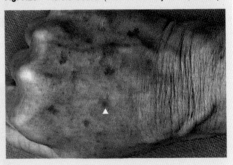

Fig. 7.27 Solar Lentigo. (From Klatt, 2022.)

Epidermoid cyst (Fig. 7.28)	• Light or skin coloured • Dome-shaped papule or nodule • May express yellowish 'cheesy' keratin via central punctum

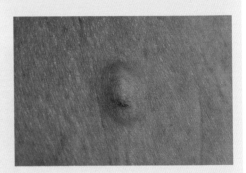

Fig. 7.28 Epidermoid cyst. (From Brinster et al., 2011.)

Considerations When Examining Darker Skin[11,12] (Figs 7.29 and 7.30)

General assessment	• Four pigments contribute to skin colour: melanin, carotene, oxygenated haemoglobin and reduced haemoglobin
	• Of these, the size, shape and location of melanin contribute most significantly to overall colour
	• Skin appears darker the nearer melanin is to the surface
	• Need to be holistic in order to consider cultural factors when exposing skin
	• Consider specific characteristics of hair and skin (i.e. damage to Afro-Caribbean by hair products)
	• Texture and temperature of skin
	• Diagnosis of some conditions can be more challenging in darker skin (i.e. rashes in septicaemia)
	• Consider comparing unaffected (normal) areas with those changing
Normal changes	• Dark skin contains more pigment with normal variations that can include 'demarcation lines', changes in nail (dark bands in the nail plate) and oral pigmentation or midline hypopigmentation (see example image below)
	• Lesions that appear red or brown on light skin can appear darker (black or purple) on dark skin
Caution regarding treatments	• Some products (i.e. steroids) may have a more dramatic effect in terms of hypopigmentation (i.e. steroids) or hyperpigmentation (i.e. oestrogens)
Primary conditions	• May be more pronounced on dark skin, i.e. vitiligo/albinism
Secondary conditions	• May develop more pronounced changes in response to underlying conditions, i.e. post-inflammatory hypopigmentation or hyperpigmentation (i.e. related to atopic eczema or acne)

Considerations When Examining Darker Skin[11,12] – cont'd

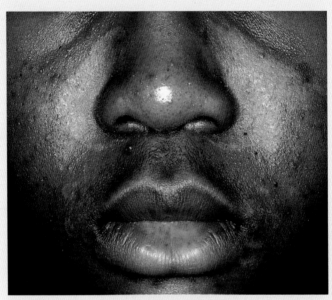

Fig. 7.29 Post-inflammatory hypopigmentation following seborrheic dermatitis. (From Paller & Mancini, 2011.)

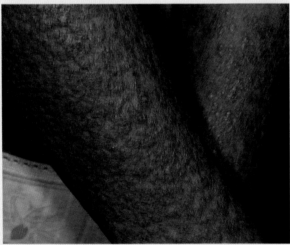

Fig. 7.30 Hyperpigmentation associated with lichenification following chronic atopic dermatitis. (From Paller & Mancini, 2016.)

Abscess

Classic history	• Localised painful swelling
	• Fluctuant vs indurated
	• If complicated:
	  • Pyrexia
	  • Local/surrounding redness/warmth/tracking
	  • Fevers and rigors

Classic findings	• Local fluctuant swelling (or indurated) • Local extension – warmth, erythema, tracking
Important differential diagnoses	• Complicated abscess • DVT • Sarcoma
UUC investigations	• FBC • CRP • Lactate • Blood cultures • Higher level: • US/CT if complicated

UUC interventions and disposal	• Incision and drainage with appropriate analgesia if:
	  • Localised, fluctuant, larger
	• Refer for specialist incision and drainage if:
	  • Face, breast, perineum, paediatric
	• Antibiotics if:
	  • Surrounding or spreading infection, indurated
	• Refer if:
	  • Systemically unwell including pyrexia, tachycardia, rigors
	  • Secondary to drug misuse
	  • Extensive/ progressive cellulitis

Special considerations	• In case of recurrence consider:
	  • Hidradenitis suppurativa
	  • Diabetes
	  • IBD
	  • Malignancy

Cellulitis

Classic history	• Red, warm skin • Sometimes painful and swollen • Skin break/port of entry
Classic findings	• As above, skin red, poorly defined margins • Pyrexia
UUC investigations	• FBC • CRP • Lactate • Blood culture • Swab culture
UUC interventions and disposal	• Systemically well – oral antibiotics • Systemically unwell – admit • Moderate peri-orbital cellulitis no visual concerns – oral antibiotics, safety net • Significant cellulitis around eye/face – IV antibiotics, admit ophthalmology • Manage underlying issues, i.e. diabetes, eczema, oedema • Consider re-assessing, serial CRP

Ear, Nose and Throat

2WW – Head and Neck – NICE Guidelines[13]

- Laryngeal cancer:
  - Consider a 2WW referral for people aged 45 and over with:
    - Persistent unexplained hoarseness, or
    - An unexplained lump in the neck
- Oral cancer:
  - Consider a 2WW referral for people with either:
    - Unexplained ulceration in the oral cavity lasting for more than 3 weeks or
    - A persistent and unexplained lump in the neck
  - Consider a 2WW referral for assessment for possible oral cancer for people who have either:
    - A lump on the lip or in the oral cavity or
    - A red or red and white patch in the oral cavity consistent with erythroplakia or erythroleukoplakia
- Thyroid cancer:
  - Consider a 2WW referral for people with an unexplained thyroid lump

General Guidelines – Respiratory Tract Infections and Antibiotics[14]

Background	• Most people develop an acute RTI every year • Major complication rates are low • No convincing evidence that lower rates of prescribing are associated with higher rates of complications • Patients who receive antibiotics typically attribute symptom resolution to this, antibiotics, and thus maintain a cycle of 'medicalising' self-limiting illness • Antibiotic resistance strongly related to antibiotic use • Difficulty for prescribers lies in identifying small number of patients who will suffer severe and/or prolonged illness or develop complications

General Guidelines – Respiratory Tract Infections and Antibiotics[14]

Strategies	• Offer no (or delayed) antibiotics to:
	  • Acute otitis media
	  • Acute sore throat/acute pharyngitis/acute tonsillitis
	  • Common cold
	  • Acute rhinosinusitis
	  • Acute cough/acute bronchitis
	• Depending on clinical assessment of severity, consider immediate antibiotic prescribing to:
	  • Bilateral acute otitis media in children younger than 2 years
	  • Acute otitis media in children with ear discharge
	  • Acute sore throat/acute pharyngitis/acute tonsillitis when three or more Centor criteria are present
	• For all antibiotic prescribing strategies advise the following average total length of the illness:
	  • Acute otitis media: 4 days
	  • Acute sore throat/acute pharyngitis/acute tonsillitis: 1 week
	  • Common cold: 1{1/2} weeks
	  • Acute rhinosinusitis: 2{1/2} weeks
	  • Acute cough/acute bronchitis: 3 weeks
	• When 'no antibiotic prescribing' strategy is adopted, offer:
	  • Reassurance that antibiotics are not needed immediately because they are likely to make little difference to symptoms and may have side effects, e.g., diarrhoea, vomiting and rash
	  • A clinical review if the condition worsens or becomes prolonged
	• When the 'delayed antibiotic' strategy is adopted, offer:
	  • Reassurance that antibiotics are not needed immediately because they are likely to make little difference to symptoms and may have side effects, e.g., diarrhoea, vomiting and rash
	  • Advice about using the delayed prescription if symptoms are not starting to settle in accordance with the expected course of the illness or if a significant worsening of symptoms occurs
	• Advice about re-consulting if there is a significant worsening of symptoms despite using the delayed prescription

Identifying complications risk	• Only offer immediate antibiotic prescription and/or further appropriate investigation and management to both adult and child patients if the patient:
	  • Is systemically very unwell
	  • Has symptoms and signs suggestive of serious illness and/or complications, particularly:
	    • Pneumonia
	    • Mastoiditis
	    • Peritonsillar abscess
	    • Peritonsillar cellulitis
	    • Intra-orbital and intracranial complications
	  • Is at high risk of serious complications because of pre-existing comorbidity including those with:
	    • Significant heart, lung, renal, liver or neuromuscular disease
	    • Immunosuppression
	    • Cystic fibrosis
	    • Young children who were born prematurely
	  • Is older than 65 years with acute cough and two or more of the following criteria, or older than 80 years with acute cough and one or more of the following criteria:
	    • Hospitalisation in previous year
	    • Type 1 or type 2 diabetes
	    • History of congestive heart failure
	    • Current use of oral glucocorticoids

Bell Palsy

Classic history	• Sudden onset unilateral facial weakness – cannot close eyes, show teeth/blow out cheeks
	• Sometimes preceding earache
	• Altered taste
	• Hyperacusis
Classic findings	• Isolated lower motor neurone facial palsy (i.e. no sparing of forehead) (Fig. 7.31)
Important differential diagnoses	• CVA
	• TIA
	• Deep parodic tumour
	• Lyme disease (exposure history, rash, joint pains)
	• Otitis media
	• Ramsay Hunt syndrome (herpes zoster causing acute facial weakness, rash in ear, palate, pharynx, face, neck or trunk)
	• Sarcoidosis
	• Guillain-Barré syndrome
	• HIV infection
	• Multiple sclerosis
	• Brain tumour
	• Horner syndrome
UUC interventions and disposal	• Prednisolone: 60 mg OD for 5/7, then 10 mg less each day
	• Antiviral medication probably not helpful
	• Artificial tears
	• Eye patch at night
	• F/u with GP/ENT
	• D/w ophthalmology if cancer regarding eye complication including trauma/ulceration

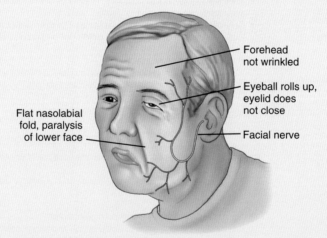

Fig. 7.31 The facial characteristics of Bell palsy. (From Shiland, 2019.)

Forehead not wrinkled

Eyeball rolls up, eyelid does not close

Facial nerve

Flat nasolabial fold, paralysis of lower face

Sudden-Onset Hearing Loss

Important differential diagnosis	• Sensorineural hearing loss • Otitis media • Otitis externa • Impacted ear wax • Tympanic membrane perforation • Ossicular dislocation • CVA • Head trauma • Autoimmune diseases • Medication • Neurological including multiple sclerosis • Meniere disease
History and characteristics	• Side/degree of hearing loss • Pain • Discharge (otorrhea) • Tinnitus • Vertigo • Swelling and local discomfort

Special considerations	• Sudden onset of hearing loss refers to hearing loss that has developed over 3 days or less
	• Adults with sudden onset of hearing loss should be referred as follows:
	  • If the hearing loss developed suddenly (over 3 days) within the past 30 days, refer immediately (to be seen within 24 h) to an ENT service or an emergency department
	  • If the hearing loss developed suddenly more than 30 days ago, refer urgently (to be seen within 2 weeks) to ENT
	• Important urgent care considerations:
	  • Adults with sudden onset of hearing loss in one or both ears that is not explained by external or middle ear causes should be referred for immediate or urgent specialist medical care
	  • Adults with rapid worsening of hearing loss in one or both ears that is not explained by external or middle ear causes should be referred for urgent specialist medical care
	• Consider urgent specific referral pathways if:
	  • Considering CVA
	  • Hearing loss in immunocompromised and have otalgia with otorrhoea that has not responded to treatment within 72 h
	  • Adults of Chinese or south-east Asian family origin who have hearing loss and a middle ear effusion not associated with an upper respiratory tract infection
	  • Any of:
	    • Unilateral or asymmetric hearing loss as a primary concern
	    • Hearing loss that fluctuates and is not associated with an upper respiratory tract infection
	    • Hyperacusis
	    • Persistent tinnitus that is unilateral, pulsatile, has significantly changed in nature or is causing distress
	    • Vertigo that has not fully resolved or is recurrent
	    • Hearing loss that is not age related

Classic Ear Images

Normal tympanic membrane
(Fig. 7.32)

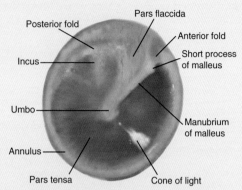

Fig. 7.32   Normal tympanic membrane. (From Jarvis, 2015.)

Acute otitis media (Fig. 7.33)

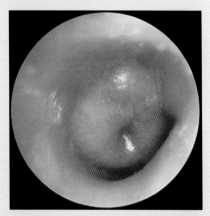

Fig. 7.33   Acute otitis media with inflamed, bulging tympanic membrane due to pus in the middle ear. (From Raftery, Lim & Ostor, 2014.)

Chronic otitis media (Fig. 7.34)

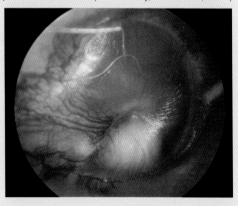

Fig. 7.34   Chronic otitis media. (From Damjanov & Linder, 1999.)

Classic Ear Images

Perforated tympanic
  membrane (Fig. 7.35)

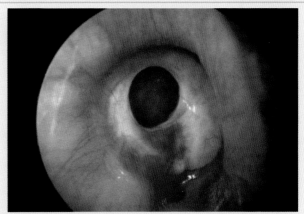

Fig. 7.35   Perforated tympanic membrane. (From Mir, 2003.)

Acute otitis externa (Fig. 7.36)

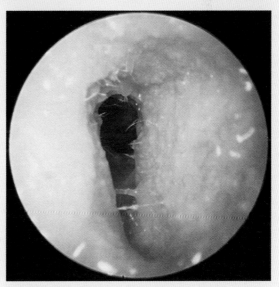

Fig. 7.36   Acute otitis externa. (From Swartz, 2014.)

Classic Ear Images – cont'd

Acute otitis externa – external changes (Fig. 7.37)

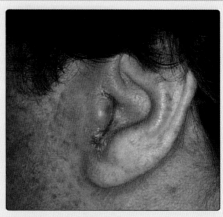

Fig. 7.37 Acute otitis externa – external changes. (From Dhillon & East, 2012.)

Otitis Externa

Classic history	• Itching
	• Pain
	• Discharge
	• Reduced hearing
Classic findings	• Inflamed, swollen canal
	• Debris/discharge
	• TM 'normal'
Important differential diagnoses	• Eczema
	• Neoplasm
UUC investigations	• Swab for MC&S
UUC interventions and disposal	• Topical antibiotics/steroids
	• Refer for aural toilet if severe
	• Admit if:
	• Concerns of malignant otitis externa
	• Extensive cellulitis
Special considerations	• 'Malignant otitis externa':
	• Involves osteomyelitis of skull base
	• Can involve facial palsy

Otitis Media

Classic history	• Fever, deafness, irritability, lethargy especially in children
	• Pain which can be relieved with 'bursting' of TM
	• Discharge if perforated
Classic findings	• Inflamed TM
	• Loss of light reflex
	• Perforation
	• Purulent discharge

Otitis Media

Important differential diagnoses	• Acute mastoiditis • Cholesteatoma • Barotrauma

UUC interventions and disposal	• Oral analgesia
	• Antibiotics may be justified if:
	  • Ongoing symptoms $\geq$4 days
	  • <2 years with bilateral infection
	  • Ear discharge
	  • Systemically unwell
	  • Recurrent infections
	• Decongestants
	• NICE recommends treatment for under 18s[15]:
	  • First line: amoxicillin
	  • Alternative: clarithromycin/erythromycin
	  • Second line: co-amoxiclav

Special considerations	• Becomes chronic suppurative otitis media if discharge >1 month (need to consider cholesteatoma)

Sinusitis

Classic history	• Nasal discharge, blocking or congestion • Facial or dental pain/pressure often worse bending forwards • Foul smell • Reduced sense of taste and smell • Associated URTI symptoms – cough, sore throat, temperature
Important differential diagnoses	• Dental pain • TMJ dysfunction • Neuralgia (including trigeminal) • Migraine • GCA • Neoplasm
UUC investigations	• Higher level: • CT if complicated/systemic concerns

UUC interventions and disposal	• Shorter illness (10 days or less):
	  • Advice
	  • Analgesia/antipyretics
	• Longer illness (>10 days) options include:
	  • Nasal steroid spray
	  • Consider antibiotics (limited data to support)
	• Worsening advice (consider other diagnoses)

Special considerations	• A bacterial infection is more likely if:
	  • Long course (>10 days)
	  • Purulent nasal discharge
	  • Severe localised pain
	  • Pyroxia
	  • Marked deterioration

TMJ Dysfunction

Classic history	• Pain: often in front of tragus, radiates to ear/temple/cheek/jaw
	• Joint noise: clicking, popping, grinding
	• Jaw locking
	• Non-specific features:
	  • Earache
	  • Tinnitus
	  • Headaches
	  • Associated/underlying stress/anxiety/depression

Important differential diagnoses	• Dental pain • Otitis media • Otitis externa • Neuralgia • Shingles • Mastoiditis • Parotitis • GCA

UUC interventions and disposal	• Initial conservative and medical options:
	  • Soft food, gently stretch and mobilise jaw
	  • Avoid extreme opening
	  • NSAIDs
	• Follow up with GP if ongoing

Tonsillitis

Classic history	• Sore throat • Malaise • Pyrexia • Dysphagia • Neck swelling and tenderness • Earache • Headache
Classic findings	• Enlarged, inflamed tonsils (Fig. 7.38) • Exudate • Tender lymph nodes • Bad breath • Pyrexia

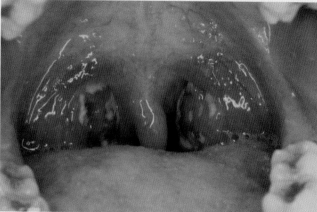

Fig. 7.38 Tonsillitis involving enlarged, inflamed tonsils with exudate. (From Neville, Damm, Allen & Bouquot, 2009.)

Tonsillitis (Fig. 7.39)

Important differential diagnoses	• Quinsy • Glandular fever • Diphtheria • Agranulocytosis • Pharyngitis • Retropharyngeal abscess • Epiglottitis • Peritonsillar abscess • Kawasaki disease • Primary HIV • Candidiasis

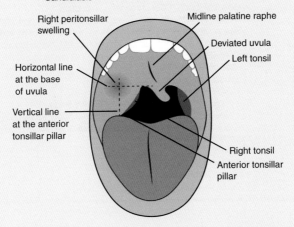

Fig. 7.39 Right-sided quinsy. (From De & Anari, 2018.)

UUC investigations	• Possibly:
	  • Throat swabs
	  • FBC
	  • Paul-Bunnell monospot test (glandular fever)

UUC interventions and disposal
Special considerations
	• Analgesia
	• Antibiotics according to scores below
	• Centor criteria:
	  • Tonsillar exudate
	  • Tender anterior cervical lymphadenopathy or lymphadenitis
	  • History of fever (over 38°C)
	  • Absence of cough
	  • Each Centor criteria score 1 point (max 4)
	  • Score of 0, 1 or 2: associated with 3%–17% likelihood of isolating streptococcus
	  • Score of 3 or 4: associated with 32%–56% likelihood of isolating streptococcus[16]
	• FeverPAIN criteria[17]:
	  • **F**ever (during previous 24 h)
	  • **P**urulence (pus on tonsils)
	  • **A**ttend rapidly (within 3 days after onset of symptoms)
	  • Severely **I**nflamed tonsils

Tonsillitis — cont'd

- No cough or coryza (inflammation of mucus membranes in the nose)
  - Each FeverPAIN criteria score 1 point (max 5)
  - Higher scores suggest more severe symptoms and likely bacterial (streptococcal) cause
  - Score of 0 or 1: associated with 13%–18% likelihood of isolating streptococcus
  - Score of 2 or 3: associated with 34%–40% likelihood of isolating streptococcus
  - Score of 4 or 5: associated with a 62%–65% likelihood of isolating streptococcus
- Management:
  - Score of 4 or 5: Offer immediate antibiotics
  - People systemically very unwell, have symptoms and signs of a more serious illness or condition, or are at high-risk of complications: Offer immediate antibiotics or further appropriate investigation and management
  - Consider referral to hospital if symptoms and signs of acute sore throat associated with any of:
    - Severe systemic infection
    - Risk of immunosuppression
    - Risk of dehydration or inability to take fluids
    - Severe suppurative complications (such as quinsy [peri-tonsillar abscess] or cellulitis, parapharyngeal or retropharyngeal abscess
- Complications include:
  - Quinsy
  - Acute otitis media
  - Acute nephritis
  - Acute rheumatism

Vertigo

Important differential diagnoses	• BPPV • Meniere disease • Vestibular neuronitis • TIA • Labyrinthitis • CVA • Acoustic neuroma • Cerebellar tumour • MS

History – characteristics	• Timing, frequency and duration:
	  • Seconds: BPPV
	  • Hours: Meniere disease
	  • Weeks: Vestibular neuronitis, labyrinthitis, post trauma
	• What is happening at time – i.e. standing up
	• Provoking or aggravating factors
	• Pain
	• Nausea
	• Neurologic symptoms
	• Hearing loss
	• Palpitations

Examination considerations	• Full ENT including tuning fork • Cranial nerves • Gait test/Romberg's • Dix-Hallpike manoeuvre

Vertigo	

Special considerations	• Dix-Hallpike manoeuvre:
	  • Inform patient that he/she cannot drive afterwards
	  • Caution if significant IHD, MSK, arthritis, etc.
	  • Seat upright
	  • Turn head 30–45 degrees to the side being tested
	  • Keep the patient's eyes focused on your eyes
	  • Hold patient's head and lie them back down with head overextended past horizontal
	  • Observe eyes for torsional nystagmus for up to 30 s
	  • Slowly return patient to sitting position
	  • Repeat both sides
	• Interpretation:
	  • Suggests BPPV if horizontal nystagmus with a latent period
	  • Suggests central cause if vertical nystagmus without a latent period

Benign Paroxysmal Positional Vertigo	
Classic history	• Recurrent short-lasting vertigo provoked by certain changes in head position including bending over, rolling over, looking up and down • Associated nausea • Poor balance
Classic findings	• Positive Dix-Hallpike
Important differential diagnoses	• Meniere disease • Vestibular neuronitis • TIA • Labyrinthitis • CVA • Acoustic neuroma • Cerebellar tumour • MS • Panic disorder

UUC interventions and disposal	• Options include:
	  • Reassurance: most improve within months
	  • Avoid provoking activities
	  • Medication: antiemetic (stemetil, cyclizine), vestibular sedative (cinnarizine, betahistine)
	  • Epley manoeuvre

End-of-Life Care[18]

Palliative Care General Principles

Good palliative care is not just about supporting someone in the last months, days and hours of life, but about enhancing the quality of life for patients and those close to them at every stage of the disease process from diagnosis onwards.

A palliative care approach should be considered alongside active disease management from an early stage in the disease process.

Palliative care focuses on the person, not the disease, and applies a holistic approach to meeting the physical, practical, functional, social, emotional and spiritual needs of patients and carers facing progressive illness and bereavement.

Palliative Care General Principles (Fig. 7.40)

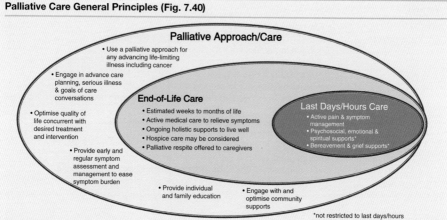

Palliative Approach/Care

- Use a palliative approach for any advancing life-limiting illness including cancer
- Engage in advance care planning, serious illness & goals of care conversations
- Optimise quality of life concurrent with desired treatment and intervention
- Provide early and regular symptom assessment and management to ease symptom burden

End-of-Life Care
- Estimated weeks to months of life
- Active medical care to relieve symptoms
- Ongoing holistic supports to live well
- Hospice care may be considered
- Palliative respite offered to caregivers

Last Days/Hours Care
- Active pain & symptom management
- Psychosocial, emotional & spiritual supports*
- Bereavement & grief supports*

- Provide individual and family education
- Engage with and optimise community supports

*not restricted to last days/hours

Fig. 7.40 Phases within the palliative care continuum. (From BC Palliative Centre for Excellence, June 26th, 2013. Updated: Interior Health, July 2019.)

Effective symptom management includes[19]:

- Evaluation: the cause of the symptom, its impact on the patient's life and the treatments tried already
- Explanation: to the patient and those close to them about the cause of the symptom and options for treating it
- Management: individualised to the particular patient. Treat any reversible causes, use non-drug treatments where available, keep drug treatment as simple as possible, seek advice when necessary
- Monitoring: review the impact of treatment regularly, paying attention to detail

Care of the Dying

Priorities	• Recognition that the person may be dying and entering the last days and hours of life • Sensitive communication between staff, the dying person and those identified as important to them • Involve the person and those identified as important to them in decisions about treatment and care to the extent that the dying person wants • Support the needs of families and others identified as important to the person including any questions or concerns they may have • Senior responsible clinician to agree a holistic individual plan of care including symptom control to be delivered
Managing symptoms	• Symptoms which may occur in the last days and hours of life include: • Pain • Nausea and vomiting • Respiratory – secretions, dyspnoea, stridor • Psycho-neurological – anxiety, panic, convulsions, delirium and terminal restlessness/agitation • Urinary incontinence/retention • Sweating • Haemorrhage

Palliative Care Emergencies – Catastrophic Haemorrhage

Classic history and findings	• Frank or occult bleeding • May be terminal event in both advanced cancer and non-malignant disease • Types: • Haemoptysis • Haematemesis • Rectal/vaginal haemorrhage • Melaena • Haematuria • Surface bleeding

Palliative Care Emergencies – Catastrophic Haemorrhage

	• Nosebleed
	• Oesophageal varices
	• Related features:
	  • Anxiety
	  • Hypotension
	  • Cool extremities
	  • Pallor
	  • Fatigue

Interventions and disposal options	• Anticipatory management for those at high risk of catastrophic haemorrhage: • Consider whether admission for urgent blood transfusion, IV fluids, etc. would be appropriate if a bleed was to occur. • Anticipatory prescribing of anxiolytic (i.e. midazolam IV, IM, buccal or sublingual but not s/c due to peripheral shut down and therefore unpredictable absorption)

Palliative Care Emergencies – Cauda Equina Compression Lumbar Spine Below L1

Classic history and findings	• Typically spinal metastases related to breast, prostate, lung cancer and myeloma • Lumbar pain with loss of power in lower limbs and loss of sphincter control • Weakness of legs, loss of lower limb tendon reflexes, sciatic pain, urinary hesitancy and peri-anal numbness
Interventions and disposal options	• Same approach as spinal cord compression

Palliative Care Emergencies – Hypercalcaemia

Classic history and findings	• Common in cancer of breast, myeloma, lung, head and neck, kidney, thyroid and cervix
	• May develop insidiously
	• Severity of symptoms are related to speed of rise of calcium
	• Common symptoms:
	  • Malaico
	  • Weakness
	  • Anorexia
	  • Thirst
	  • Nausea
	  • Constipation
	• More severe symptoms:
	  • Vomiting
	  • Ileus
	  • Delirium
	  • Seizures
	  • Drowsiness
	  • Coma
	• Pain can be precipitated or exacerbated

Interventions and disposal options	• Low threshold for checking:
	  • Corrected calcium
	  • U&Es
	  • eGFR
	  • LFTs
	• Seek immediate specialist advice

Palliative Care Emergencies – Hypercalcaemia – cont'd

Special considerations	• Definition is corrected serum calcium >2.7 mmol/L (some variation between laboratories)
	• Further treatment options depend on advice and calcium levels but may include:
	  • Whether first or recurring
	  • Prognosis and prior quality of life
	  • Patient consent to IV treatment and tests
	  • Medication changes
	  • IV fluids
	  • IV bisphosphonate

Palliative Care Emergencies – Metastatic Spinal Cord Compression

Classic history and findings	• Affects 5%–10% of patients with cancer
	• Most common in prostate, lung and breast cancer, myeloma
	• Symptoms may be vague, needs high index of suspicion:
	  • Back/spinal pain, may radiate in a radicular 'band-like' pattern
	  • Progressive or unremitting
	  • May be worse on coughing or straining, prevent sleep or be absent
	  • Nerve root pain in limbs
	  • Weakness of limbs (out of proportion to general condition of patient)
	  • Difficulty walking
	  • Sensory changes – tingling, numbness
	  • Difficulty passing urine (usually late presentation)
	  • Constipation or faecal incontinence
	  • Absent or increased reflexes
	  • Extensor plantars, clonus
	  • Distended bladder

Interventions and disposal options	• Urgent same-day assessment by specialist team • Commence high-dose steroids (PPI cover) immediately if there is clinical suspicion, even if diagnosis not confirmed • Urgent MRI of whole spine scan (within 24 h) • Immobilisation for patients with symptoms and signs suggestive of spinal instability and spinal cord compression

Special considerations	• Catastrophic event – aim is to prevent establishment of paresis.
	• Patients with cancer and neurological signs or symptoms of spinal cord compression should be treated as an oncological emergency
	• Early treatment aims to:
	  • Prevent permanent paralysis, loss of bowel and bladder control, loss of independence and quality of life
	  • Maximise recovery of neurological function
	  • Provide local tumour and pain control

Palliative Care Emergencies – Neutropenic Sepsis

Classic history and findings	• Consider in any patient who has had recent chemotherapy who is deteriorating, especially if it is unexpected
	• Most likely 7–10 days after treatment, but can be up to 1 month
	• Early signs:
	  • Flu-like symptoms
	  • Temperature of 38°C or above
	  • Rigors
	• Late signs:
	  • Anxiety
	  • Confusion
	  • Cold and clammy
	  • Hypotension, tachycardia
	  • Diarrhoea
	• NSAIDs and paracetamol affect temperature so may mask condition/sepsis

Palliative Care Emergencies – Neutropenic Sepsis

Interventions and disposal options	• If condition suspected, DO NOT DELAY • P1 transfer, liaise with acute oncology team • Meanwhile treat as sepsis
Special considerations	• Life-threatening event, needs urgent treatment irrespective of life expectancy

Palliative Care Emergencies – Superior Vena Cava Obstruction

Classic history and findings	• Commonest causes (95%) are lung cancer and non-Hodgkin lymphoma • Swelling of face, neck, arms • Headache • Dizziness • CNS depression • Seizures • Dyspnoea • Dilated veins – neck, trunk, arms • Hoarse voice • Stridor
Interventions and disposal options	• Admit unless in the last days of life, in which case seek specialist advice • Sit patient up • Oxygen if hypoxic • Dexamethasone 16 mg oral/13.2 mg SC once daily • Consider Furosemide 40 mg IV or oral • Seek specialist oncological advice for ongoing management

Special considerations	• Involves compression/invasion or thrombosis of superior vena cava due to tumour or nodal mass within mediastinum
	• Further interventions may include:
	  • Endo-venous stent
	  • Thrombolysis
	  • Radiotherapy and/or chemotherapy
	• Overall prognosis is poor
	• Without treatment, SVCO may cause death within a few days
	• Even with treatment, 1-year survival is 17%

Palliative Care Symptom Management – Anorexia

Assessment	• Causes:
	  • Paraneoplastic effect of cancer
	  • Impaired gastric emptying
	  • Medication – e.g. opioids, NSRIs
	  • Poor oral hygiene, candidiasis
	  • Altered taste or smell
	  • Anxiety, depression, delirium
	  • Any of the causes of nausea

Management approach	• Treat reversible causes
	• Explain an effect of cancer itself
	• Listen to fears and anxieties (failure to eat can cause fear and conflict)
	• Dietary advice:
	  • Eat energy-rich foods such as full fat milk, yoghurt and spreads
	  • Food fortification, e.g. add cream to soups, butter to vegetables
	  • Encourage snacking and more frequent small portions
	  • Avoid excessive amounts of food
	  • Consider dietician unless prognosis short

Palliative Care Symptom Management – Anorexia – cont'd

- Pharmacological management:
  - Corticosteroid: short-term improvement of appetite. Rapid effect but tends to decrease after 3–4 weeks, may also help reduce nausea, improve energy and general feeling of wellbeing
  - Consider need for gastric protection
  - Dexamethasone – 2–6 mg orally once daily in the morning; assess after 1 week; if beneficial, continue – reduce weekly to lowest effective dose; if no benefit after 1 week, then stop; side effects: fluid retention, candidiasis, myopathy, insomnia, gastritis and steroid-induced diabetes
  - Prokinetic: if impaired gastric emptying suspected, metoclopramide 10 mg three times a day
  - Seek specialist advice if no response

Palliative Care Symptom Management – Anxiety

Assessment	• Number of associated causes including uncertainty about the future, separation from loved ones, financial, work and social worries as well as unrelieved pain or other symptoms
	• May be new to the individual, but is commoner in patients with pre-existing anxiety disorders
	• Symptoms and signs of anxiety may be due to or exaggerated by organic problems such as:
	• Hypoxia
	• Sepsis
	• Medications (e.g. antipsychotics; SSRIs; steroids)
	• Drug or substance withdrawal (e.g. benzodiazepines/opioids/nicotine/ alcohol)
	• Metabolic causes (e.g. hypoglycaemia/ thyrotoxicosis)
	• Poorly controlled pain/other symptoms
	• Dementia
Management approach	• Severity of underlying disease and the overall prognosis guides management decisions
	• Treat contributing factors such as pain and other symptoms, hypoxia, sepsis, etc.
	• If prognosis >4 weeks, use non-pharmacological measures and follow NICE guideline for management of generalised anxiety disorder and panic disorder
	• If prognosis <4 weeks, some non-pharmacological measures can still be helpful, but use of benzodiazepines may also be considered particularly if anxiety is severe
	• Non-pharmacological measures:
	• Acknowledge and discuss anxiety and specific fears as well as patient's own views and understanding
	• Distraction
	• Relaxation techniques
	• Counselling
	• Cognitive behavioural therapy (CBT)
	• Consider involvement of local psychological or psychiatric services
	• Self-help (e.g. 'bibliotherapy' – use of written material)
	• Support groups
	• Day hospice if appropriate
	• Assess how family coping
	• Pharmacological:
	• If prognosis <4 weeks: benzodiazepines
	• If prognosis >4 weeks: SSRI ± benzodiazepines

Palliative Care Symptom Management – Breathlessness

Assessment	• Common in patients with advanced disease, tends to become more common and severe in the last few weeks of life
	• Breathlessness caused by respiratory depression needs to be managed by specific medications, i.e. naloxone
	• Unpleasant subjective sensation that does not always correlate with clinical pathology
	• Patient's distress indicates severity
	• Causes usually multi-factorial: physical, psychological, social and spiritual factors all contribute to subjective sensation
	• Important to recognise and treat potentially reversible causes of breathlessness
	• Assessment:
	  • History and clinical examination
	  • Investigations, e.g. chest x-ray

Management approach	• Treat reversible causes
	• General approach:
	  • Cardiac failure and pulmonary oedema: diuretics/ACE inhibitors/nitrates/opioids
	  • Pneumonia: antibiotics where appropriate
	  • Bronchospasm: bronchodilators ± steroids
	  • Anaemia: transfusion for symptoms rather than haemoglobin level
	  • Pulmonary embolism: anticoagulation
	  • Anxiety: anxiolytics
	  • Superior vena cava obstruction: see above, high-dose steroids, referral for radiotherapy/chemotherapy/stent
	  • Tracheal/bronchial obstruction: referral to oncologist for radiotherapy/stenting
	  • Lung metastases: referral to oncologist for radiotherapy/chemotherapy
	  • Pleural effusion/pericardial effusion/ascites: consider drainage procedures
	• Non-pharmacological measures:
	  • Reassure and explain
	  • Distract, relaxation techniques
	  • Position patient to aid breathing
	  • Increase air movement – fan/open window
	  • Physiotherapy – decrease respiratory secretions and breathing exercises
	  • Occupational therapy – modify activities of daily living to help symptoms
	  • Establish meaning of breathlessness for patient and explore fears
	  • Psychological support, reduce distress of anxiety and depression
	• Pharmacological:
	  • Opioids (decrease perception of breathlessness, decrease anxiety and decrease pain)
	  • Benzodiazepines (do not relieve breathlessness have a role when anxiety exacerbates breathlessness, contraindicated unless patient is imminently dying in acute severe pulmonary insufficiency, untreated sleep apnoea syndrome, severe hepatic impairment and myasthenia gravis, used with caution in patients with type 2 respiratory failure)
	  • SSRI (if prognosis >4 weeks)
	  • Corticosteroids may reduce inflammatory oedema
	  • Oxygen therapy:
	    • Limited evidence but may help dyspnoeic patients who are hypoxic (SaO_2 <92%) at rest or who become so on exertion
	    • For patients with COPD who are chronically hypoxic do not use more than 28% oxygen
	    • Oxygen therapy may lead to limited mobility, barrier to communication, inconvenience and cost implications
	    • Safety implications include fire risk from smoking (including e-cigarettes) or other heat sources such as radiators, matches or lit candles
	  • Nebulised medications (sodium chloride 0.9% or Salbutamol nebules), need to monitor the first dose for adverse effects and stop after 3 days if no response

Palliative Care Symptom Management – Constipation

Assessment	• Causes:
	  • Drug induced
	  • Dehydration
	  • Reduced mobility (access to toilet, privacy)
	  • Altered dietary intake
	  • Hypercalcaemia
	  • Neurological
	  • Gastrointestinal obstruction
	• History – past and present bowel habit, use of laxatives, date of last bowel action, current medication, other causative factors
	• Abdominal palpation and auscultation, digital rectal examination
	• Investigations – if needed for treatment, e.g. abdominal x-ray, calcium levels
	• For intractable constipation, seek specialist advice

Management approach	• Prevention is key
	• Consider stimulant laxatives for all on opioid with aim of achieving a regular bowel movement without straining every 1–3 days
	• Encourage good oral fluid and dietary intake, including fruit and fruit juice
	• Use oral laxatives first line
	• Approximately one-third of palliative care patients need rectal measures, either because of failed oral treatment or electively (should be avoided, where possible, in patients who are neutropenic or thrombocytopenic, because of the risk of infection or bleeding)
	• Laxative choices:
	  • Soft bulky stools/low colonic activity: oral stimulant, i.e. bisacodyl, senna, sodium picosulfate
	  • Colon full, no colic: stimulant ± softening agent, i.e. senna + docusate sodium
	  • Colon full and colic present: macrogols, i.e. movicol, laxido
	  • Hard dry faeces: softening agents, i.e. docusate sodium, arachis oil enema (avoid if known nut allergy)
	  • Hard faeces, full rectum/colon: stimulant plus softener, e.g. bisacodyl tablets or senna plus docusate sodium or second-line macrogols, i.e. movicol, laxido or third line – Glycerol 4 g suppository and Bisacodyl 10 mg suppository or, if ineffective, sodium citrate enema
	  • Faecal impaction: arachis oil retention enema (avoid if known nut allergy) ± phosphate enema or second-line macrogols, i.e. movicol, laxido
	  • Opioid-induced constipation resistant to the above methods: seek specialist advice

Palliative Care Symptom Management – Cough

Assessment	• May be cancer-related/treatment-related or due to other diseases • May serve a physiological purpose and therefore where possible expectoration/physiotherapy should be encouraged
Management approach	• Malignancy related: consider referral to oncologist for radiotherapy/chemotherapy/laser therapy or corticosteroids • Treatment related: medication review, e.g. ACE inhibitor-induced cough • Cardiac failure and pulmonary oedema: diuretics/ACE inhibitors • Pneumonia: antibiotics if appropriate • Asthma and COPD: bronchodilators ± steroids • Reduce sputum viscosity: carbocisteine • Infection: physiotherapy/nebulised sodium chloride 0.9% antibiotics, maintain hydration • Recurrent laryngeal nerve palsy: consider ENT referral • Pleural effusion: drainage

Palliative Care Symptom Management – Delirium and Confusion

Assessment	• Characterised by 4 core features:
	  • Disturbance of consciousness and attention
	  • Change in cognition, perception and psychomotor behaviour
	  • Develops over short period of time and fluctuates during day
	  • The direct consequence of a general medical condition, drug withdrawal or intoxication
	• Can have acute or sub-acute onset (sub-acute seen commonly in the elderly) and should be distinguished from dementia
	• Validated tools to detect delirium include the 4AT and the CAM
	• Types of delirium:
	  • Hyperactive delirium – predominantly restless and agitated
	  • Hypoactive delirium – predominantly drowsy and inactive (often overlooked and symptoms may be mistaken for depression or dementia)
	  • Mixed motor type – with evidence of both hyperactive and hypoactive symptoms in the past 24 h
	• Can be a great source of distress to patients and carers and is associated with higher mortality
	• Causes can be multi-factorial so assessment is essential
	• Use of the mnemonic PINCHME is helpful in remembering possible reversible causes of delirium
	  • Pain
	  • Infection
	  • Nutrition
	  • Constipation
	  • Hydration and hypoxia
	  • Medication and metabolic
	  • Environment

Management approach	• Non-pharmacological:
	  • Provide environmental and personal orientation
	  • Manage patient in a quiet well-lit room
	  • Support and correct any sensory deprivation (use of glasses/hearing aids, etc.)
	  • Ensure continuity of care
	  • Maintain hydration
	  • Hallucinations, vivid dreams and misperceptions may reflect unresolved fears and anxieties
	  • Reassure relatives and carers that the patient's confusion is secondary to a physical condition and provide information about how they can best help the person
	• Specific causes:
	  • Drug related (opioids, corticosteroids, sedatives, antimuscarinics): reduce or stop suspected medication or switch to suitable alternative
	  • Withdrawal (alcohol, nicotine, benzodiazepines, opioids): possibly allow patient to continue to use responsible agent. Nicotine patches may be useful
	  • Metabolic (respiratory failure, liver failure, renal failure, hypoglycaemia, hyperglycaemia, hypercalcaemia, adrenal, thyroid or pituitary dysfunction, infection, nutrition): treat reversible causes, consider oxygen
	  • Raised intracranial pressure: dexamethasone, specialist advice
	  • Other (dehydration, shock, anaemia, pain, constipation, urinary retention, sleep, environment): treat reversible causes if possible and appropriate (e.g. IV fluids, transfusion, manage pain/constipation/catheterise)
	• Pharmacological:
	  • Evidence for the role of antipsychotics in managing delirium symptoms is variable – only use if symptoms are marked, persistent and causing distress to the patient and non-pharmacological interventions have not worked
	• Choices of medication:
	  • Delirium where sedation undesirable: start with haloperidol, consider benzodiazepine if alcohol withdrawal is suspected
	  • Agitated delirium where sedation would be beneficial: olanzapine or levomepromazine (more sedating)
	  • Acutely disturbed, violent or aggressive, at risk to themselves or others: haloperidol and seek advice from mental health crisis team

Palliative Care Symptom Management – Diarrhoea

Assessment	• Establish cause
	• Review diet (some gastrostomy feeds cause diarrhoea)
	• Seek dietitian advice if required
	• Review medication
	• Clinical assessment including rectal examination and inspection of stool
	• Exclude:
	  • Infective cause
	  • Constipation/faecal impaction with overflow (plain abdominal x-ray if overflow may help if suspected – treat as for constipation)
	  • If in the last days of life, treat symptomatically, do not investigate

Management approach	• Cause:
	  • Drugs (laxatives, magnesium antacids, PPI, NSAID): review medication and stop if possible
	  • Antibiotics (altered bowel flora): stop antibiotic if possible, stool sample to exclude *Clostridium difficile*
	  • Infection: fluid and electrolyte support, stool sample for culture – treat with appropriate drug for identified bacteria
	  • Overflow (constipation, partial obstruction): identify, treat underlying constipation, soften stool if partial obstruction, avoid specifically constipating treatments
	  • Acute radiation enteritis/chemotherapy/secretory diarrhoea (e.g. AIDS, tumour, fistula): seek oncology advice
	  • Surgical resection (stomach, ileal, colon), bile salt diarrhoea: cholestyramine (on specialist advice)
	  • Steatorrhoea: pancreatic enzyme ± PPI (reduces gastric acid destruction of enzymes)
	• Using loperamide and codeine
	• Give loperamide 2 mg after each loose stool, max 16 mg a day
	• If not controlling diarrhoea, rapidly change to 2 mg four times a day then 4 mg four times a day if required
	• Substitute codeine 30 mg four times a day orally if ineffective
	• Thereafter consider a combination of loperamide + codeine and seek specialist advice

Palliative Care Symptom Management – Fatigue

Assessment	• Causes:
	  • Underlying disease process (e.g. cancer or as a consequence of treatment
	  • Anaemia: consider blood transfusion if appropriate
	  • Dehydration: consider IV/SC hydration
	  • Pain: optimise pain control
	  • Iatrogenic: opioids, benzodiazepines, post chemotherapy
	  • Poor nutrition: consider dietician referral, build up drinks
	  • Depression: consider antidepressants
	  • Endocrine abnormalities: consult with endocrinologist
	  • Often combination of reversible and irreversible causes

Management approach	• Consider reversible causes
	• Non-pharmacological:
	  • Paced exercise programme
	  • Cognitive behavioural therapy
	  • Mindfulness programme
	  • Acupuncture
	• Pharmacological management
	  • Corticosteroids: reduces effect of pro-inflammatory cytokines and improves general feeling of wellbeing (dexamethasone 4–8 mg orally once daily in the morning for a maximum of 14 days)

Palliative Care Symptom Management – GI Obstruction

Assessment	• Occurs in approximately 3% of all cancer patients
	• More frequent complication if advanced intra-abdominal cancer (e.g. colon −10%; ovary −25%)
	• Site of obstruction: small bowel in 50%; large bowel in 30%; both in 20%
	• Mechanical or functional cause(s) – often more than one
	• May be partial or complete
	• Onset may be over hours or days; initial intermittent symptoms may worsen and become continuous, or may resolve spontaneously (usually temporarily)
	• Signs and symptoms include:
	  • Nausea and vomiting (earlier and more profuse in higher obstruction)
	  • Pain due to abdominal colic or tumour itself
	  • Abdominal distension (especially distal obstruction)
	  • Altered bowel habit (from constipation to diarrhoea due to overflow)
	  • Bowel sounds (from absent to hyperactive and audible)
	• Radiology – if needed to distinguish faecal impaction, constipation and ascites
	• Rarely an emergency – take time to discuss situation with patient and family to allow them to make an informed choice about management

Management approach	• Seek specialist advice
	• May be reversible in some patients
	• Consider surgery if:
	  • Patient willing
	  • Discrete and easily reversible mechanical cause of obstruction
	  • Prognosis >12 weeks if treated
	• Poor surgical outcome likely if:
	  • Previous abdominal radiotherapy
	  • Small intestinal obstruction; multiple sites
	  • Extensive disease
	  • Poor condition
	  • Cachexia
	  • Poor mobility
	• Surgery likely contraindicated if:
	  • Carcinomatosis peritonei
	  • Findings suggest intervention is futile
	  • Poor physical condition
	  • Short prognosis <12 weeks

Palliative Care Symptom Management – Hiccups

Assessment	• Consider severity, duration and impact on a patient's quality of life
	• Causes include:
	  • Gastric stasis and distension (most common)
	  • Gastro-oesophageal reflux
	  • Metabolic disturbances (uraemia, hypercalcaemia, magnesium deficiency)
	  • Infection
	  • Irritation of diaphragm or phrenic nerve
	  • Hepatic disease/hepatomegaly
	  • Cerebral causes (e.g. tumour, metastases)
	  • Damage to phrenic nerve over its course from skull to diaphragm, e.g. shingles, pressure from mediastinal tumour

Palliative Care Symptom Management – Hiccups – cont'd

Management approach	• Often stop spontaneously
	• Treatment only required if hiccups are persistent and cause discomfort/distress
	• Try simple physical manoeuvres initially and those that have worked previously
	• Non-pharmacological management:
	  • Simple 'home remedies' (sipping iced water, swallowing crushed ice, breathing into a paper bag, holding breath, drinking from wrong/opposite side of a cup, rubbing soft palate with a swab to stimulate the nasopharynx
	  • Acupuncture
	• Pharmacological management:
	  • Gastric distension ± gastro-oesophageal reflux: peppermint water/metoclopramide/anti-flatulent, i.e. simethicone/PPI
	  • Diaphragmatic or phrenic nerve irritation > seek specialist advice, baclofen, antiepileptic, i.e. gabapentin, nifedipine, midazolam
	  • Systemic causes, e.g. biochemical, infection: treat underlying cause, seek specialist advice, haloperidol, midazolam
	  • CNS tumour, meningeal infiltration by cancer: seek specialist advice, antiepileptic, i.e. gabapentin, baclofen
	  • Hepatic, mediastinal or cerebral compression/ irritation by disease/ tumour: dexamethasone

Palliative Care Symptom Management – Insomnia

Assessment	• Assess beliefs about normal sleep and the impact of insomnia on activities and quality of life • Ask about duration of insomnia and possible contributing factors
Management approach	• Correct contributory factors where possible, e.g. pain, delirium, depression, anxiety, obstructive sleep apnoea • Non-pharmacological including general sleep hygiene measures • Pharmacological management if symptoms severe using a Z-drug or benzodiazepine with short half-life (duration should not usually exceed 4 weeks)

Palliative Care Symptom Management – Nausea and Vomiting

Assessment	• 30%–40% of patients with advanced cancer have nausea and/or vomiting • Review history, recent investigations and medication • Examine for underlying causes and likely physiological mechanisms • Only investigate if outcome will affect management

Management approach	• Reversible/treatable causes (*management in brackets*) include:
	  • Drugs (*stop or find alternative unless essential*)
	  • Uncontrolled pain (*analgesia non-oral route until vomiting settles*)
	  • Anxiety (*determine fears; explain; anxiolytic*)
	  • Cough (*suppressant*)
	  • Urinary retention (*catheterise*)
	  • Constipation (*laxatives*)
	  • Liver metastases (*corticosteroids; anticancer treatment*)

Palliative Care Symptom Management – Nausea and Vomiting

- Raised intracranial pressure *(corticosteroids, e.g. dexamethasone)*
- Electrolyte disturbances *(correct if possible and appropriate)*
- Hypercalcaemia *(rehydration and intravenous bisphosphonate)*
- Uraemia *(urinary diversion or stent)*
- Oral/oesophageal candidiasis *(antifungal such as fluconazole, nystatin, miconazole)*
- Infection *(antibiotic)*
- Gastritis *(stop irritant drug; add PPI)*
- Bowel obstruction *(see separate section below)*
- If no response, reassess cause:
  - If likely cause is unchanged – consider alternative route of administration, alternative antiemetic or broad-spectrum antiemetic
  - If likely cause has changed – try appropriate antiemetic for that cause
- May need combinations of antiemetic therapy
- If symptoms still not improving seek specialist advice

Palliative Care Symptom Management – Oral Health

Assessment	<ul><li>Assess mouth on a daily basis</li><li>Features of a healthy mouth include:<ul><li>Clean and moist with saliva</li><li>Gums, tongue and cheeks are healthy and pink</li><li>No holes in the teeth or broken fillings</li><li>Dentures clean and fit well</li><li>No mouth ulcers or undiagnosed red or white patches</li></ul></li></ul>
Management approach	<ul><li>Preventative: regular teeth and tongue cleaning and denture care, adequate oral fluid, lips should be moisturised sparingly with lip balm</li><li>Aphthous ulcers: hydrocortisone oromucosal tablet/topical analgesic gels, i.e. choline salicylate, Bonjela, lidocaine ointment/antiseptic mouthwash</li><li>Viral ulcers: acyclovir/topical gels (above)</li><li>Malignant ulcers: consider antibiotic</li><li>Radiation stomatitis: benzydamine 0.15% mouthwash or spray/mucosal protectant gel, i.e. episil, gelclair/paracetamol/opioid analgesics/seek expert advice</li><li>Gingivitis: metronidazole/antiseptic mouthwash, i.e. chlorhexidine</li><li>Dry mouth: review medications (opioids, antimuscarinics)/increase oral fluid intake/saliva substitutes/moisturising agents/boiled sweets, ice cubes, sugar free chewing gum/sodium chloride mouthwashes/sprays/nebulisers/pilocarpine (seek specialist advice)</li><li>Coated tongue: chow pineapple chunks/brush tongue with soft toothbrush</li><li>Fungal infection: nystatin oral suspension/fluconazole/miconazole</li><li>Bacterial infection: consider antibiotics</li><li>Dry lips: yellow/white soft paraffin or normal lip salve</li></ul>

Palliative Care Symptom Management – Pain

Assessment	• Ask about:
	  • Site and radiation
	  • Character
	  • Onset, intensity and severity
	  • Timing and duration
	  • Exacerbating factors
	  • Relieving factors, including medication
	  • Effect on function, sleep and mood
	  • Response to previous medication
	  • Associated symptoms
	• Examine
	• Assess impact of pain on the patient and family
	• Consider if other factors, such as emotional, psychological or spiritual distress, are affecting pain perception
	• Consider appropriate investigations to determine cause
	• Common causes of pain:
	  • Disease related: direct invasion by cancer, distension of an organ, pressure on surrounding structures
	  • Bone pain: worse on pressure or stressing bone or weight bearing
	  • Nerve pain: burning, shooting, tingling, jagging, altered sensation, dermatomal distribution
	  • Spinal cord compression: back or spinal pain in a radicular 'band-like' pattern
	  • Liver pain: hepatomegaly, right upper quadrant tenderness, referred pain in shoulder tip
	  • Raised intracranial pressure: headache, nausea or both, often worse in the morning or with lying down
	  • Colic: intermittent cramping pain. Consider bowel obstruction, bladder spasm
	  • Treatment-related: chemotherapy neuropathy, constipation due to opioids, radiation-induced mucositis
	  • Debility: pressure sores, severe cachexia, oral candidiasis
	  • Other unrelated illnesses: arthritis, osteoporosis, vascular disease, gastritis

Management approach	• Set realistic goals, e.g. pain-free overnight/at rest/on movement • Give patients and carers information and instructions about the pain and its management • Review regularly • Manage expectations regarding optimal pain management; it may not be achievable for them to be pain-free at all times • Consider checking renal and liver function before initiating analgesia if no recent blood results are available • Use the WHO Analgesic Ladder approach (Fig. 7.41)[20] (up to strong opioids) plus adjuvant analgesia if required (may include amitriptyline, gabapentin, pregabalin, duloxetine, corticosteroids, etc.)

Palliative Care Symptom Management – Pain

Treatment of cancer pain

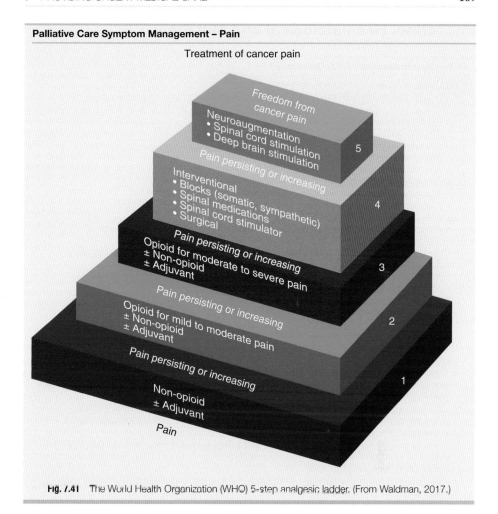

Fig. 7.41 The World Health Organization (WHO) 5-step analgesic ladder. (From Waldman, 2017.)

Palliative Care Symptom Management – Respiratory Secretions

Assessment	• Excess respiratory secretions common in patients near the end of life
	• Caused by fluid pooling in the upper airways, arising from one or more sources:
	  • Saliva (most common)
	  • Bronchial mucosa (e.g. inflammation/infection)
	  • Pulmonary oedema
	  • Gastric reflux

Management approach	• Those semiconscious or unconscious are not usually troubled by secretions • Explanation to family members important as they may find the secretions distressing, particularly if noisy rattling breathing • Position patient semi-prone, to encourage postural drainage, unless the secretions are caused by pulmonary oedema or gastric reflux when the patient should be more upright • Suction of the upper airway is usually reserved for unconscious patients, as it can otherwise be distressing • Pharmacological: Glycopyrronium or alternative antimuscarinic drugs (hyoscine butylbromide or hyoscine hydrobromide)

Endocrine, Haematological and Metabolic

2WW – Haematological – NICE Guidelines[21]

- Leukaemia in adults:
  - Consider very urgent (within 48h) full blood count in adults with any of the following:
    - Pallor
    - Persistent fatigue
    - Unexplained fever
    - Unexplained persistent or recurrent infection
    - Generalised lymphadenopathy
    - Unexplained bruising
    - Unexplained bleeding
    - Unexplained petechiae
    - Hepatosplenomegaly
- Leukaemia in children and young people:
  - Refer for immediate specialist assessment for leukaemia if unexplained petechiae or hepatosplenomegaly
  - Offer a very urgent full blood count (within 48h) in children and young people with any of the following:
    - Pallor
    - Persistent fatigue
    - Unexplained fever
    - Unexplained persistent infection
    - Generalised lymphadenopathy
    - Persistent or unexplained bone pain
    - Unexplained bruising
- Myeloma:
  - Offer full blood count, blood tests for calcium and plasma viscosity or erythrocyte sedimentation rate to assess for myeloma in people aged 60 and over with persistent bone pain, particularly back pain, or unexplained fracture
  - Offer very urgent protein electrophoresis and a Bence-Jones protein urine test (within 48h) to assess for myeloma in people aged 60 and over with hypercalcaemia or leukopenia and a presentation that is consistent with possible myeloma
  - Consider very urgent protein electrophoresis and a Bence-Jones protein urine test (within 48h) to assess for myeloma if the plasma viscosity or erythrocyte sedimentation rate and presentation are consistent with possible myeloma
  - 2WW referral if the results of protein electrophoresis or a Bence-Jones protein urine test suggest myeloma
- Non-Hodgkin lymphoma in adults:
  - Consider 2WW referral for non-Hodgkin lymphoma in adults presenting with unexplained lymphadenopathy or splenomegaly. When considering referral, take into account any associated symptoms, particularly fever, night sweats, shortness of breath, pruritus or weight loss
- Non-Hodgkin lymphoma in children and young people:
  - Consider a very urgent (within 48h) referral for specialist assessment for non-Hodgkin lymphoma in children and young people presenting with unexplained lymphadenopathy or splenomegaly. When considering referral, take into account any associated symptoms, particularly fever, night sweats, shortness of breath, pruritus or weight loss
- Hodgkin lymphoma in adults:
  - Consider a 2WW referral for Hodgkin lymphoma in adults presenting with unexplained lymphadenopathy. When considering referral, take into account any associated symptoms, particularly fever, night sweats, shortness of breath, pruritus, weight loss or alcohol-induced lymph node pain
- Hodgkin lymphoma in children and young people:
  - Consider a very urgent (within 48h) referral for specialist assessment for Hodgkin lymphoma in children and young people presenting with unexplained lymphadenopathy. When considering referral, take into account any associated symptoms, particularly fever, night sweats, shortness of breath, pruritus or weight loss

Addisonian Crisis	
Classic history	• Non-specific background features of adrenal insufficiency:
	• Weight loss and fatigue
	• Hyperpigmentation
	• Nausea, diarrhoea, vomiting
	• Apathy, irritability, depression
	• Oligomenorrhoea
	• In crisis:
	• Shock
	• Confusion
	• Weakness
	• Altered consciousness
	• Hypoglycaemia
UUC investigations	• FBC
	• U&E
	• ABG
	• BM
	• Blood glucose
UUC interventions and disposal	• May be asked to supply routine medication OOH as it is key to avoid interruption. Requests could include:
	• Hydrocortisone for glucocorticoid replacement (or longer-acting glucocorticoids, such as prednisolone and dexamethasone, to avoid peaks and troughs)
	• Fludrocortisone for mineralocorticoid replacement
	• Dehydroepiandrosterone (unlicensed) for androgen replacement
	• For crisis:
	• Arrange emergency admission if suspected
	• IV access
	• IV fluid – 1000 mL N/Saline
	• Hydrocortisone IM or IV
	• Licensing: Use Hydrocortisone sodium phosphate (Efcortesol) or Hydrocortisone sodium succinate (Solu-Cortef) but *not* hydrocortisone acetate
	• Dose:
	• Adults: 100 mg
	• Children 6 years of age or older: 50–100 mg (clinical judgement depending on the age and size of the child)
	• Children 1–5 years of age: 50 mg
	• Infants up to 1 year of age: 25 mg
	• Correct hypoglycaemia
	• IV antibiotics if appropriate

Hyperglycaemic Crisis – Diabetic Ketoacidosis	
Classic history	• Signs of dehydration: thirst, polydipsia, polyuria, decreased skin turgor, dry mouth, hypotension, tachycardia
	• GI symptoms: nausea, vomiting, abdominal pain
	• Hyperventilation: deep rapid (Kussmaul) breathing, acetone breath
	• True coma: altered unconsciousness
	• Causes (the four 'I's):
	• Infections: especially UTI, respiratory, skin
	• Infarction: cardiac, CVA, GI, peripheral vessels
	• Insufficient insulin
	• Intercurrent illness

Hyperglycaemic Crisis – Diabetic Ketoacidosis – cont'd

UUC investigations	• BM (blood glucose >11)
	• Blood glucose
	• FBC, creatinine, osmolality
	• CXR (pneumonia)
	• ECG/cardiac monitoring
	• Blood cultures
	• Urine/sputum MC&S
	• Higher level:
	  • Osmolality
	  • ABG

UUC interventions and disposal	• ABC
	• Oxygen
	• IV fluids (0.9% saline)
	• P1 transfer with pre-alert
	• Higher level:
	  • Insulin infusion
	  • Manage electrolyte imbalance
	  • NG tube
	  • Catheter
	  • Treat infection
	  • Manage clotting
	  • Admission to most appropriate area (AMU to ITU)

Special considerations	• Hyperosmolar hyperglycaemic State (HHS):
	  • Caused by intercurrent illness, poor diabetic control, dehydration
	  • Develops over days/weeks
	  • More common in elderly

Hypoglycaemia

Classic history	• Sweatiness, pallor, tachycardia, hunger, trembling, irritability, altered consciousness, irrational behaviour
	• Can mimic neurological presentations with coma, seizures, acute confusion, hemiparesis
	• Causes can include:
	  • Imbalance of medication in diabetic patient
	  • Alcohol
	  • Addison
	  • Pituitary insufficiency
	  • Post gastric surgery
	  • Liver failure
	  • Malaria
	  • Insulinomas
	  • Extra-pancreatic tumours
	  • Overdose of hypoglycaemic drugs

Classic findings	• Cognitive function can decrease if BM <3.0 mmol/L • But symptoms uncommon if BM >2.5 mmol/L
UUC investigations	• BM • Blood glucose

UUC interventions and disposal	• If BM <3.0 mmol/L, take blood glucose but start treatment without waiting for result
	• Conscious:
	  • Oral: 3–15 g fast acting oral carbohydrate
	• Unconscious:
	  • Glucagon 1 mg (SC, IM or IV)
	  • Glucose 10% IV
	• Retest BM after 15 min

Special considerations	• 90% fully recover within 20 min – if the cause is identified and fully corrected then can be discharged after period of observation • Persistent altered mental state requires ITU admission, CT scan, etc.

Hyperkalaemia

Classic history	• Often symptomatic
	• Severe hyperkalaemia:
	  • Muscular function:
	    • Paraesthesia
	    • Muscle weakness
	    • Fatigue
	  • Cardiac function:
	    • Arrhythmias
	    • Chest pain, along with sweating, nausea, vomiting, lethargy, weakness, dizziness

Classic findings	• Causes:
	  • Prolonged tourniquet time
	  • Reading error/haemolysis
	  • Trans-cellular shift:
	    • DKA/acidosis
	    • Drugs – including digoxin, succinylcholine, β-blocker
	  • Renal:
	    • Acute/chronic renal failure
	    • Renal tubular acidosis
	    • Drugs (spironolactone, amiloride, ACE inhibitors, ARB, NSAID, heparin)
	    • Mineralocorticoid deficiency
	  • Increasing circulating potassium:
	    • Supplementation
	    • Tumour
	    • Rhabdomyolysis
	    • Trauma, burns
	  • Diabetic nephropathy

UUC investigations	• Repeat U&E • ECG • Serum glucose • BM • ABG

UUC interventions and disposal	• If K+ is 5.5–5.9 mmol/L *and* no symptoms *and* eGFR stable (not decreased by >10%) *and* potassium not recent increase, then:
	  • Review/change medication
	  • F/u with GP
	  • Repeat U&Es within 2 weeks
	• If K+ is 5.5–5.9 mmol/L and other conditions above not met:
	  • Admit
	• If K+ is 6.0–7.0 mmol/L:
	  • Recheck blood
	  • ECG
	  • Admit if remains high
	• If K+ is > 6.4 mmol/L
	  • P1 transfer, admit
	• Also admit if:
	  • Feels unwell
	  • Any arrhythmia
	  • Symptomatic (weakness/paralysis/fatigue/paraesthesia)
	  • ECG changes
	  • Fall in eGFR (>10% in 1–2 weeks)
	  • Rapid increase in K+ (>0.5 mmol/L in 1–2 weeks)
	  • Underlying heart disease, cirrhosis, or kidney disease

Hyperkalaemia – cont'd

Special considerations

- Classic associated ECG changes (Fig. 7.42):
  - Tall, peaked (tented) T waves (T wave larger than R wave in more than 1 lead)
  - First degree heart block (prolonged PR interval) (>0.2 s)
  - Flattened or absent P waves
  - ST-segment depression
  - S and T wave merging (sine wave pattern)
  - Widened QRS (>0.12 s)
  - Arrythmias including bradycardia, ventricular tachycardia or fibrillation
  - Cardiac arrest (pulseless electrical activity (PEA), ventricular fibrillation/pulseless ventricular tachycardia (VF/VT), asystole)

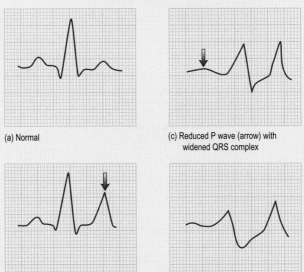

(a) Normal

(c) Reduced P wave (arrow) with widened QRS complex

(b) Tented T wave (arrow)

(d) 'Sine wave' pattern (pre-cardiac arrest)

Fig. 7.42 Progressive ECG changes with increasing hyperkalaemia. (From Kumar & Clark, 2011.)

Hypokalaemia

Classic history

- Lethargy/confusion
- Muscle wasting
- Weakness
- Paralysis, fasciculations, tetany, spasms especially extensor muscle spasms of hands and feet
- Paraesthesia of hands and feet
- Nausea
- Vomiting
- Abdominal distension
- Polyuria

Hypokalaemia

Classic findings	• Consider causes including:
	  • Anorexia/starvation
	  • Diuretics
	  • Loss:
	    • Faecal – colitis, laxative abuse
	    • Vomit – due to any cause
	    • Skin – burns, excessive sweating
	  • Excessive alcohol intake
	  • Process which stimulates uptake of potassium from the extracellular fluid into cells:
	    • Intravenous insulin for treatment of hyperglycaemia (in particular, diabetic ketoacidosis)
	    • Stimulation of sympathetic β2 receptors (e.g., with high-dose salbutamol)
	  • Verapamil overdose
	  • Small cell lung cancer
	  • After vitamin B12 or folate replacement in megaloblastic anaemia

UUC interventions and disposal	• K+ is 3.1–3.5 mmol/L:
	  • Compare trend
	  • Check/change medications
	  • Sando K: 2 tabs OD until K+>3.5 mmol/L
	  • Inform/f/u with GP
	  • Consider ECG if higher risk
	• K+ is 2.6–3.0 mmol/L:
	  • Compare trend
	  • Repeat if possibly unreliable
	  • ECG
	  • Consider A&E if rapid change (>0.3 mmol/L in 2–3 days) or high risk
	  • Check/change medications
	  • Sando K: 2 tabs bd or TDS until K+>3.5 mmol/L
	  • Inform/f/u with GP
	• K+ is < 2.6 mmol/L
	  • Compare trend
	  • Urgent repeat sample and ECG
	  • Refer urgently to A&E

Special considerations	• ECG changes include (Fig. 7.43):
	  • Flattened/inverted T waves
	  • ST segment depression
	  • Prolonged QT interval
	  • Tall U waves
	  • Atrial arrythmias
	  • Ventricular tachycardia or ventricular fibrillation and torsade de pointes

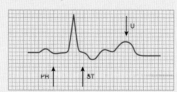

Fig. 7.43 ECG changes related to hypokalaemia. (From Adappa & Hewitt, 2022.)

Hypernatraemia

Classic history	• Thirst
	• Confusion
	• Coma
	• If severe – cerebral haemorrhage or thrombosis
	• Causes:
	  • Diabetes insipidus
	  • Diarrhoea
	  • Vomiting
	  • Diuretics
	  • Cushing
	  • Conn syndrome
	  • Iatrogenic

UUC investigations	• Repeat U&E • Glucose • Higher level: • Serum and urine osmolality

UUC interventions and disposal	• Admit if:
	  • Na >155 mmol/L
	  • Na 146–155 mmol/L and unable to drink or neurology
	  • Hyperosmolar hyperglycaemic state (HSS) (hypernatraemia and hyperglycaemia >20 mmol/L)
	• If Na <155 mmol/L:
	  • Increase daily fluids
	  • Daily U&E
	  • Avoid rapid NA reduction to prevent cerebral oedema

Hyponatraemia

Classic history	• Definition is plasma sodium < 135 mmol/L
	• Often initially non-specific
	• Range from lethargy and anorexia to agitation, disorientation, seizures and coma
	• Mild hyponatraemia: serum sodium concentration 130–135 mmol/L
	• Moderate hyponatraemia: serum sodium concentration 125–129 mmol/L
	• Severe hyponatraemia: serum sodium concentration less than 125 mmol/L
	• Symptoms may vary:
	• Mild or chronic hyponatraemia (without exacerbation) may produce no symptoms
	• Moderate hyponatraemia:
	  • Headache, nausea, vomiting
	  • Malaise, irritability, depression, personality change
	• Severe hyponatraemia,
	  • Confusion, drowsiness, convulsions
	  • Diminished reflexes, extensor plantar response
	  • Cheyne-Stokes respiration
	  • Coma, death
	• Ask about:
	  • Previous similar readings
	  • Neurological features
	  • Fluid balance information
	  • Volume status (dehydrated, oedema)
	  • Medical, drug, smoking history

Hyponatraemia

UUC investigations	• Repeat U&E
	• Glucose
	• Higher level:
	  • Serum osmolality
	  • Urine osmolality and sodium
	  • Ca, Mg, Phosphate
	  • TFTs
	  • Cortisol (short synacthen test)

UUC interventions and disposal	• If encephalopathy:
	  • Admit
	• Without encephalopathy:
	  • Slowly correct

Special considerations	• Main causes: • Hypovolaemia: GI tract (D&V) or kidneys (renal dx, diuretics, Addison) • Water gain: excessive drinking, SIADH, hyperglycaemia, ecstasy, recreational drugs, polydipsia • Hypervolaemia: nephrotic syndrome, cardiac failure, ascites • Drugs

Thyrotoxic Crisis

Classic history	• CVS: palpitations, tachycardia, AF
	• Neurological: irritability, emotional lability, coma
	• General: high temperature, weight loss, increased appetite, tremor, heat intolerance, sweating, itch
	• Causes:
	  • Imbalance of thyroid treatment
	  • Thyroid surgery or radio-iodine treatment
	  • Intercurrent infection (especially respiratory)
	  • Trauma
	  • Emotional stress
	  • DKA, hyperosmolar crisis, insulin-induced hypoglycaemia
	  • Pre-eclampsia

Important differential diagnosis	• Acute pulmonary oedema • Neuroleptic malignant syndrome • Septic shock • Anticholinergic/sympathomimetic OD • Drug withdrawal • Acute anxiety

UUC investigations	• FBC
	• U&E
	• ABG
	• BM
	• Blood glucose
	• CXR (infection, CHF)
	• ECG (arrhythmias)
	• Higher level:
	  • Serum thyroxine
	  • T3
	  • Calcium

UUC interventions and disposal	• Oxygen • IV access • Fluid: 0.9% saline • Consider sedation with diazepam PO/IV/haloperidol • Oral dexamethasone/hydrocortisone IV • Broad spectrum antibiotic if relevant • Admit – higher level treatment needed

Neutropaenia

Classic findings	• Mild: 1.0–2.5 × 10⁹/L
	• Moderate: 0.5–1.0 × 10⁹/L
	• Severe: <0.5 × 10⁹/L
Important differential diagnosis	• Viral infection (including glandular fever)
	• Autoimmune (including rheumatoid arthritis, SLE)
	• Splenomegaly
	• Drugs (various)
	• Haematological (leukaemia, lymphoma, myelodysplasia, B12 and folate deficiency)
UUC investigations	• If <1.0 × 10⁹/L:
	• Repeat test
	• If second test <1.0 × 10⁹/L: then admit
	• If second test >1.0 × 10⁹/L: then see own GP for f/u tests including film, ANA, LDH, B12, folate, protein electrophoresis
	• If >1.0 × 10⁹/L:
	• If well and FBC normal: then see own GP for f/u tests including film, ANA, LDH, B12, folate, protein electrophoresis
	• If well and FBC abnormal: discuss with o/c haematologist, may need admission
	• If febrile or unwell: urgent admission

Lymphocytosis

Classic history	• Check if recent viral infection or smoking/chronic inflammatory condition
Classic findings	• Lymphocyte count >5 × 10⁹/L
UUC interventions and disposal	• GP f/u for repeat FBC, blood film, mono spot test if well
	• Urgent referral if:
	• Hb <100 and/or platelets <100 × 10⁹/L
	• B symptoms (fever, night sweats, weight loss)
	• Unexplained pyrexia >38°C for >2 weeks
	• Lymphadenopathy
	• Hepato- or splenomegaly
	• Extreme fatigue

Thrombocytopaenia

Classic history	• May be asymptomatic
	• Bruising
	• Bleeding (various including nosebleeds, menorrhagia, bowel, urine)
	• Fatigue
Classic findings	• Bruising/purpura/petechiae
	• Enlarged spleen
Important differential diagnosis and causes	• Decreased platelet production:
	• Anaemias
	• Leukaemia and other cancers
	• Myelodysplasia
	• Infections including measles, hepatitis C or HIV
	• Metastatic cancer
	• B12 and folate deficiency
	• Chemotherapy, radiotherapy
	• Alcohol

Thrombocytopaenia

	• Increased platelet destruction:
	  • Pregnancy
	  • Auto-immune including lupus and rheumatoid arthritis
	  • Sepsis
	  • thrombotic
	  • Haemolytic uraemic syndrome
	  • Medications including heparin, quinine, sulfa-containing antibiotics, anticonvulsants
	  • Thyroid disorders
	  • Disseminated intravascular coagulopathy

UUC investigations	• FBC (consider rechecking) • Lactate • CRP

UUC interventions and disposal	• Urgent referral if:
	  • Platelets $<50 \times 10^9$/L
	  • Platelets <100 and Hb <100
	  • Neutrophils $<1 \times 10^9$/L
	  • Splenomegaly
	  • Lymphadenopathy
	  • Pregnant

Thrombocytosis

Classic history	• To consider:
	  • Splenectomy
	  • Blood loss
	  • Inflammatory disorder
	  • Chronic infection
	  • Thrombosis
	  • Occult malignancy

Classic findings	• Splenomegaly • Evidence inflammation/infection/malignancy

Important differential diagnosis and causes	• Primary (bone marrow disorders)
	  • Essential thrombocythemia
	  • Polycythaemia vera
	  • Myelofibrosis
	  • Chronic myeloid leukaemia
	  • Myelodysplastic syndrome
	• Secondary or reactive
	  • Malignancy
	  • Infection (acute or chronic)
	  • Inflammatory disorders (i.e. inflammatory bowel disease, arthritis, connective tissue disorders)
	  • Blood loss (acute or chronic)
	  • Post trauma, surgery, chemotherapy
	  • Splenectomy/hyposplenism

UUC interventions and disposal	• Consider risk of malignancy
	• Thrombus formation is extremely rare (unless pat count $>1000 \times 10^9$/L plus other risk factors for thrombosis), complications of the underlying cause more common
	• Persistent thrombocytosis (platelets $>450 \times 10^9$/L over 2–3 months) requires:
	  • Full history and examination
	  • FBC
	  • Ferritin/iron studies
	  • CRP/ESR
	  • Autoantibody screen, rheumatoid factor (if inflammatory disease suspected)

Gastroenterology and General Surgery

2WW – UPPER GI – NICE Guidelines[22]

- Oesophageal cancer:
  - Offer urgent direct access (within 2 weeks) to people:
    - With dysphagia or
    - Aged 55 and over with weight loss and any of the following:
      - Upper abdominal pain
      - Reflux
      - Dyspepsia
  - Consider non-urgent direct access upper gastrointestinal endoscopy to assess for oesophageal cancer in people with haematemesis
  - Consider non-urgent direct access upper gastrointestinal endoscopy to assess for oesophageal cancer in people aged 55 or over with:
    - Treatment-resistant dyspepsia or
    - Upper abdominal pain with low haemoglobin levels or
    - Raised platelet count with any of the following:
      - Nausea
      - Vomiting
      - Weight loss
      - Reflux
      - Dyspepsia
      - Upper abdominal pain, or
    - Nausea or vomiting with any of the following:
      - Weight loss
      - Reflux
      - Dyspepsia
      - Upper abdominal pain
- Pancreatic cancer:
  - 2WW referral for people who are aged 40 and over and have jaundice
  - Consider an urgent direct access CT scan (to be performed within 2 weeks), or an urgent ultrasound scan if CT is not available, to assess for pancreatic cancer in people aged 60 and over with weight loss and any of the following:
    - Diarrhoea
    - Back pain
    - Abdominal pain
    - Nausea
    - Vomiting
    - Constipation
    - New-onset diabetes
- Stomach cancer:
  - Consider 2WW referral for people with an upper abdominal mass consistent with stomach cancer
  - Offer urgent direct access upper gastrointestinal endoscopy (to be performed within 2 weeks) to assess for stomach cancer in people:
    - With dysphagia or
    - Aged 55 and over with weight loss and any of the following:
      - Upper abdominal pain
      - Reflux
      - Dyspepsia
    - Consider non-urgent direct access upper gastrointestinal endoscopy to assess for stomach cancer in people with haematemesis
  - Consider non-urgent direct access upper gastrointestinal endoscopy to assess for stomach cancer in people aged 55 or over with:
    - Treatment-resistant dyspepsia or
    - Upper abdominal pain with low haemoglobin levels or
    - Raised platelet count with any of the following:
      - Nausea

2WW – UPPER GI – NICE Guidelines[22]

- Vomiting
- Weight loss
- Reflux
- Dyspepsia
- Upper abdominal pain, or
- Nausea or vomiting with any of the following:
  - Weight loss
  - Reflux
  - Dyspepsia
  - Upper abdominal pain
- Gall bladder cancer:
  - Consider an urgent direct access ultrasound scan (to be performed within 2 weeks) to assess for gall bladder cancer in people with an upper abdominal mass consistent with an enlarged gall bladder
- Liver cancer:
  - Consider an urgent direct access ultrasound scan (to be performed within 2 weeks) to assess for liver cancer in people with an upper abdominal mass consistent with an enlarged liver

2WW – LOWER GI – NICE Guidelines[23]

- Colorectal cancer:
  - 2WW referral if
    - Aged 40 and over with unexplained weight loss and abdominal pain or
    - Aged 50 and over with unexplained rectal bleeding or
    - Aged 60 and over with:
      - Iron-deficiency anaemia or
      - Changes in their bowel habit, or
      - Tests show occult blood in their faeces
  - Consider 2WW referral for adults with a rectal or abdominal mass
  - Consider 2WW referral for adults aged under 50 with rectal bleeding and any of the following unexplained symptoms or findings:
    - Abdominal pain
    - Change in bowel habit
    - Weight loss
    - Iron-deficiency anaemia
  - Faecal Immunological Testing (FIT): above recommendation has been replaced by our diagnostics guidance on 'FIT' testing. The diagnostics guidance recommends tests for occult blood in faeces, for people without rectal bleeding but with unexplained symptoms that do not meet the criteria for a suspected cancer pathway referral in recommendations
- Anal cancer:
  - Consider 2WW referral for people with an unexplained anal mass or unexplained anal ulceration

Acute Appendicitis

Classic history	• Central, colicky abdominal pain which migrates to RIF/McBurney point • Vomiting • Pyrexia • Loss of appetite • Altered bowel habit • Sometimes testicular pain

Acute Appendicitis – cont'd

Classic findings	• Ranges from normal to severe shock • Tenderness McBurney point ± peritonitis • Guarding, rebound tenderness • PR: tenderness high right • RIF mass – possible abscess • Retrocaecal appendicitis – psoas and obturator signs
Relevant anatomy	• McBurney point
Important differential diagnoses	• See list in 'Acute Abdominal Pain' table

UUC investigations	• BM
	• Urinalysis
	• Pregnancy test
	• FBC
	• U&E
	• LFT
	• Amylase
	• GGT
	• CRP
	• Lactate
	• ECG (ACS)
	• CXR (basal pneumonia)
	• AXR (if thinking obstruction, perforation, ureteric calculi)
	• Higher level especially for atypical cases:
	  • CT
	  • USS

UUC interventions and disposal	• IV fluids • Analgesia • Antiemetic • IV antibiotics if delayed surgery • Surgical referral

Acute Cholecystitis

Classic history	• RUQ pain • Radiating to right side back • Vomiting • Fever • Pale stools • Dark urine
Classic findings	• RUQ tenderness especially on inspiration (Murphy sign) • Common bile duct stones: • Biliary obstruction with jaundice, pale stools, dark urine
Important differential diagnoses	• See list in 'Acute Abdominal Pain' table

UUC investigations	• BM
	• Urinalysis
	• Pregnancy test
	• FBC
	• U&E
	• LFT
	• Amylase
	• GGT
	• CRP
	• Lactate
	• ECG (ACS)
	• CXR (basal pneumonia)
	• AXR (if thinking obstruction, perforation, ureteric calculi)
	• Higher level:
	  • USS
	  • MR cholangiopancreatography
	  • CT
	  • HIDA scanning (cholescintigraphy or hepatobiliary scintigraphy)

Acute Cholecystitis

UUC interventions and disposal	• IV analgesia • Antiemetic • IV antibiotics • IV fluids
Special considerations	• May present as an acute or chronic (i.e. known gallstones) condition; if pain resolves and there are no residual features or signs then discharge for GP follow-up. • Courvoisier's Law: If jaundiced and gallbladder is palpable, then unlikely to be a stone (consider neoplasm) • Ascending cholangitis: 'Charcot triad' of abode pain, jaundice and fever – may be very unwell, resuscitate for septic shock

Acute Pancreatitis

Classic history	• Severe constant epigastric pain • Radiation to centre of back • Nausea and vomiting
Classic findings	• Distress • Sweating, pyrexia • Shocked • Epigastric tenderness • Decreased bowel sounds • Jaundice (obstruction) • 'Gray-Turner sign' – flank bruising • 'Cullen sign' – periumbilical bruising
Important differential diagnoses	• See list in 'Acute Abdominal Pain' table
UUC investigations	• BM • Urinalysis • Pregnancy test • FBC • U&E • LFT • Amylase • GGT • CRP • Lactate • ECG (ACS) • CXR (basal pneumonia) • AXR (if thinking obstruction, perforation, ureteric calculi) • Higher level: 　• Abdominal USS 　　• Magnetic resonance cholangiopancreatography
UUC interventions and disposal	• Oxygen • IV fluids • IV analgesia • Antiemetic • NG tube • Catheter • P1 transfer, pre-alert
Special considerations	• Significant mortality and complication rate

Constipation

Classic history

- Infrequent (abnormal) passing of stool which may be harder and difficult to pass
- Abdominal pain and bloating/distension
- Possibly overflow diarrhoea
- Can describe using Bristol stool chart (Fig. 7.44)

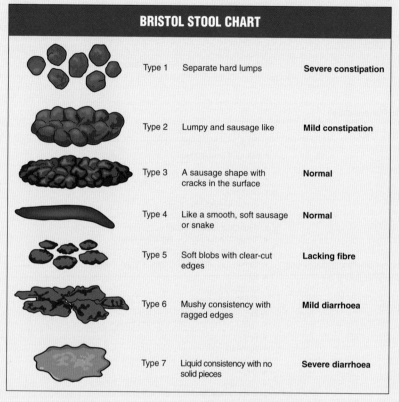

BRISTOL STOOL CHART

Type 1	Separate hard lumps	**Severe constipation**
Type 2	Lumpy and sausage like	**Mild constipation**
Type 3	A sausage shape with cracks in the surface	**Normal**
Type 4	Like a smooth, soft sausage or snake	**Normal**
Type 5	Soft blobs with clear-cut edges	**Lacking fibre**
Type 6	Mushy consistency with ragged edges	**Mild diarrhoea**
Type 7	Liquid consistency with no solid pieces	**Severe diarrhoea**

Fig. 7.44 The Bristol stool chart. (Wikimedia Commons: File: BristolStoolChart.png (website), https://commons.wikimedia.org/wiki/File:BristolStoolChart.png, Updated June 18, 2018.)

Classic findings

- Mild tenderness
- Left sided faecal loading
- PR: may or not identify faecal material

Important differential diagnosis

- Consider underlying causes which include:
  - Dehydration
  - Drugs (especially opiates)
  - Behavioural including in response to painful anal conditions
  - Bowel motility and megacolon
  - Neoplasm
  - Metabolic imbalance
  - Diverticular disease
  - Spinal cord problems
  - Irritable bowel syndrome
  - Hypothyroidism

Constipation

UUC investigations	• Dependant on cause, may include:
	  • AXR
	  • U&Es
	  • FBC
	  • Higher:
	    • Calcium
	    • TFTs

UUC interventions and disposal	• Consider primary causes
	• Advice – diet, exercise, hydration
	• Short term laxatives:
	  • First: bulk-forming laxative (Ispaghula, methylcellulose, sterculia)
	  • Next: add or switch to an osmotic laxative (macrogols, phosphate and sodium citrate enemas) then lactulose
	  • If stools soft but difficult to pass, or there is a sensation of inadequate emptying, add a stimulant laxative (senna, bisacodyl and sodium picosulfate, docusate)
	  • If opioid-induced constipation:
	  • Don't prescribe bulk-forming laxatives
	  • Offer osmotic laxative and stimulant laxative (or docusate)
	• If faecal impaction then consider:
	  • Phosphate enema
	  • Movicol in adults

Special considerations	• Consider as part of red flag cancer assessment
	• Very common in children who may present with:
	  • Overflow diarrhoea
	  • Non-specific abdominal pain
	  • Irritability
	  • Malaise
	  • Pain on defection and subsequent behavioural changes
	• In elderly consider if:
	  • Confusion or delirium, functional decline
	  • Nausea or loss of appetite
	  • Overflow diarrhoea
	  • Urinary retention

Diverticulitis

Classic history	• LIF discomfort • Altered/loose bowels • Low-grade pyrexia • Occasional large rectal bleed • Or, if complicated: • Acute abdomen, fistulas, faecal peritonitis
Classic findings	• Low grade fever • LIF tenderness • Rigidity, rebid tenderness, guarding • Consider sepsis
Important differential diagnoses	• See list in 'Acute Abdominal Pain' table
UUC investigations	• See list in 'Acute Abdominal Pain' table

Diverticulitis – cont'd

UUC interventions and disposal	• Analgesia
	• If 'well' and diagnosis clear:
	  • Oral antibiotics
	  • Analgesia
	• If 'unwell'/complicated, then treat as acute abdomen including IV fluids, antibiotics, refer general surgery

Gastroenteritis

Classic history	• Diarrhoea • Vomiting
Classic findings	• Abdominal tenderness • Pyrexia • Dehydration: from thirst, dry mouth to shock/drowsiness
Important differential diagnoses	• Poor diet • Food allergy • Food poisoning • Salmonellosis • Ulcerative colitis • Crohn disease • Appendicitis • Otitis media (in children) • Urinary tract infection • Typhoid/paratyphoid • Intussusception • Neurological causes of vomiting • Pre-eclampsia
UUC investigations	• Often none • Otherwise, based on related concerns: • FBC, U&E, CRP, lactate, AXR
UUC interventions and disposal	• Most are self-limiting • Refer/admit babies <3/12 • Oral rehydration therapy • Antiemetic • Antibiotics only for specific illness after testing
Special considerations	• Notifiable disease • Rare in fully breast-fed infants • Public Health England directs that those with gastroenteritis should be considered potentially infectious to others and excluded from work, school, social settings, etc. until a minimum of 48 h symptom free

Gastrointestinal Bleed – Lower

Important differential diagnoses	• Upper GI bleed • Angiodysplasia • Diverticular disease • Neoplasm • IBD • Infection • Haemorrhoids • Anal fissure • Meckel diverticulum • Alternative source – ENT, respiratory

Gastrointestinal Bleed – Lower

History and characteristics	• Nature • Volume • Duration • Colour • Mucus • Stool characteristics • Syncope • Other bleeds, bruises • Drug, alcohol history
Examination considerations	• ABC • Assess shock/hypovolaemia • Pallor • CRT • Observations • GCS • Abdominal tenderness, masses • DRE
Potential investigations	• FBC • Clotting • U&E • Glucose • Group and save (secondary care upwards)

Special considerations	• Risk of mortality and complications increases with:
	  • Age
	  • Comorbidity
	  • Shock
	  • NSAID use
	• Treatment may include:
	  • ABC
	  • Oxygen
	  • Large bore cannula
	  • Fluid (later blood, FFP, clotting factors)
	  • Catheter
	  • NG tube
	  • Prophylactic antibiotics

GI Bleed – Upper

Important differential diagnoses	• Peptic ulceration (duodenal, gastric) • Inflammation (oesophagitis, gastritis) • Varices • Neoplasm • Bleeding diathesis • Mallory-Weiss tear • Pancreatitis • Nasal bleed
History and characteristics	• Haematemesis • PR bleed/melaena • Duration • Amount • Abdominal pain • Past history • Weight loss • Family history • Bruising, other bleeding • Syncope • Drug, alcohol, smoking

GI Bleed – Upper – cont'd

Examination considerations	• ABC • Assess shock/hypovolaemia • Pallor • CRT • Observations • GCS • Abdominal tenderness, masses • DRE

Potential investigations	• FBC
	• Clotting
	• U&E
	• Glucose
	• Higher level:
	  • Group and save (secondary care upwards)
	  • Endoscopy
	  • FIT (faecal immuno-chemical testing)

Special considerations	Various scores (Glasgow-Blatchford bleeding score, Rockall Score, AIMS65 score) differently predict risk in various ways including in-hospital mortality, length of stay, costs, inpatient mortality, transfusion requirements, rebleeding and delayed (6 month) mortality.[24] The Glasgow-Blatchford score specifically:
	• Identifies low-risk patients who might be suitable for outpatient management
	• Risk of mortality and complications increases with:
	  • Age
	  • Comorbidity
	  • Liver disease
	  • Continued bleeding
	  • Elevated urea
	  • PR bleeding
	• Treatment may include:
	  • ABC
	  • Oxygen
	  • Large bore cannula
	  • Fluid (later blood, FFP, clotting factors)
	  • Catheter
	  • Prophylactic antibiotics

Haemorrhoids

Classic history	• Bright red rectal bleed • Blood on paper not in stools • Local pain/discomfort/swelling • Pruritus ani
Important differential diagnoses	• IBD • Polyp • Rectal prolapse • Rectal carcinoma • Anal wart • Fissure • Tear
UUC investigations	• Abdominal examination • DRE

Haemorrhoids

UUC interventions and disposal	• Check abdomen, examine anus • If no prolapsed/external pile then digital rectal examination and surgical follow-up • Prolapsed pile: good analgesia, rest, stool softeners • Thrombosed external pile: conservative management with good analgesia, sometimes I&D by surgeons
Special considerations	• Diagnosis may be confirmed by proctoscopy, sigmoidoscopy

Hernia

Classic history	• New, persistent or intermittent lump/swelling
	• Ache, 'dragging'
	• If complications (incarceration/strangulation):
	  • Fixed, tender
	  • Obstruction (vomiting, distension)

Classic findings	• Simple: reducible, cough impulse • Incarceration: tender, irreducible, local warmth. signs of obstruction

Important differential diagnoses	• Dependant on site of hernia may include:
	  • Lipoma
	  • Lymphadenopathy
	  • Testicular origin (hydrocele, varicocele)

UUC interventions and disposal	• Simple:
	  • GP follow-up with advice regarding incarceration
	• If incarcerated:
	  • Emergency surgical review
	  • Consider 'drip and suck' meanwhile (nasogastric tube, intravenous fluids)
	  • Analgesia

Intestinal Obstruction

Classic history	• Abdominal pain (often colic)
	• Distension
	• Vomiting
	• Constipation
	• Causes:
	  • Adhesions
	  • Obstructed hernia
	  • Neoplasm
	  • Volvulus
	  • Inflammatory mass, i.e. diverticular disease and Crohn
	  • Peptic ulcer disease
	  • Gallstone Ileus
	  • Intussusception

Classic findings	• Dehydration • Distension • Old surgical scars • Resonant percussion • 'Tinkling' or absent bowels sounds • PR: empty rectum
Important differential diagnoses	• See list in 'Acute Abdominal Pain' table

Intestinal Obstruction – cont'd	
UUC investigations	• See list in 'Acute Abdominal Pain' table
	• AXR: may show distended lops of bowel, fluid levels
UUC interventions and disposal	• 'Drip & suck'
	• IV fluids
	• Oxygen
	• IV analgesia including morphine
	• IV antiemetic
	• NG tube
	• Refer to surgical team
Special considerations	• Depending on cause, initial treatment may be medical if no peritonism

Peptic Ulcer	
Classic history	• Epigastric pain which can spread to rest of abdomen
	• Worse on coughing or moving
	• Radiates to shoulder tip
	• 'Indigestion'
Classic findings	• Patient 'lies still' or writhes in pain
	• Absent bowel sounds
	• Shock
	• Peritonitis
	• Fever
Important differential diagnoses	• See list in 'Acute Abdominal Pain' table
UUC investigations	• See list in 'Acute Abdominal Pain' table
	• Erect CXR shows air under diaphragm
UUC interventions and disposal	• Oxygen
	• IV fluids
	• IV analgesia, antiemetic
	• IV antibiotics
Special considerations	• Role of *Helicobacter Pylori* testing

Mental Health

General Considerations[42]	
Mental state examination	• Appearance (dress, clean, shaven, well kempt, posture, gait)
	• Behaviour (facial expression, cooperation vs aggression, calm vs agitation, activity, agitation, level of arousal, physiology including flushed, etc.)
	• Speech (form and pattern, volume and rate, coherence, logic, 'pressure')
	• Mood (apathy, irritability, pessimism vs optimism, high vs low mood, deliberate self-harm ideation)
	• Thought (delusions, unusual beliefs or ideas, paranoia, preoccupations, irrationality, potential for safety concerns)
	• Perception (unusual sensations or hallucinations (visual, auditory, touch, taste, smell)
	• Intellect (cognitive function, orientation)
	• Insight: (attribution and explanation of symptoms)

General Considerations[42] – cont'd

Recognising mental health emergencies
- Situations requiring urgent interventions include:
  - Extreme mania
  - Nihilism
  - Self-neglect
  - Suicidal ideation
  - Sexual exploitation
  - Safeguarding considerations
  - Risky and threatening behaviour

Acute Distress Including Bereavement

Classic history and findings
- Responses to stressful experiences (including bereavement) may include:
  - Distress
  - Panic
  - Tearfulness
  - Low mood
  - Anger and irritability
  - Poor sleep and appetite
- Varies between individuals and cultures
- Consider 'cycle' or stages of bereavement

Interventions and disposal options
- Acknowledge as normal human experience and response
- Potentially very short-term hypnotics
- Referral including CRUSE bereavement counselling service
- Rarely antidepressants for those developing longer term depressive features

Mental Health 'Crisis'

Classic history and findings
- Overwhelming by events
- New or linked to preceding mental ill health
- More common in those with severe mental illness and personality disorder
- Usual coping mechanisms fail
- May involve decompensation/maladaptive coping strategies such as substance abuse, deliberate self-harm, violent behaviour, panic attacks, disabling anxiety, suicidal ideation

Interventions and disposal options
- Depends on scale of complaint and risk assessment
- May involve:
  - Acknowledgement and support
  - Counsellor and mental health team referral
  - Crisis team referral
  - Admission

Depression and Suicidal Ideation

Classic history and findings
Core features of depression include:
- Sustained low mood
- Anhedonia
- Poor or increased sleep
- Poor or increased appetite
- Poor concentration and ability to prioritise
- Psychomotor agitation or retardation
- Reduced libido

Depression and Suicidal Ideation – cont'd

Interventions and disposal options	• Long-term treatment plans should be made by the patient's GP where options include:
	  • Mild/recent onset depressive symptoms: close active monitoring, individual guided self-help (based on CBT principles), structured group physical activity programmes
	  • Past history of moderate or severe depression, subthreshold depressive symptoms (that have been present for at least 2 years), subthreshold depressive symptoms or mild depression that persist(s) after other interventions: consider antidepressants
	  • Moderate or severe depression: antidepressant medication, high intensity psychological interventions
	• More urgent interventions depend on assessment of risk of suicide and self-harm, in which case discuss with crisis team

Special considerations	• Risk factors for suicide include:
	  • Male
	  • Older
	  • Single
	  • Isolation
	  • Previous suicidal ideation
	  • Marked depressive symptoms
	  • Alcohol and drug misuse
	  • Longstanding mental illness
	  • Painful or disabling physical illness
	  • Recent psychiatric inpatient treatment
	  • Self-discharge against medical advice
	  • Previous impulsive behaviour, including self-harm
	  • Some careers including farmers, vets, emergency workers
	  • Ongoing legal or criminal proceedings
	  • Family, personal or social disruption including separation from loved ones

Severe Behaviour Change

Classic history and findings	• Acute, extreme change in behaviour • Aggression, irritability, outbursts, screaming, shouting, threats to self or others

Differential diagnosis	• Psychiatric:
	  • Anxiety
	  • Panic disorder
	  • Mania
	  • Schizophrenia and other psychotic disorders
	  • Personality disorder
	  • Situational stressors
	• Acute confusional state
	• Intoxication (drugs and alcohol)
	• Brain injury
	• Non-medical including anger, frustration, criminal behaviour

Severe Behaviour Change

Interventions and disposal options	• Consider safety of you and others • Involve police, security where necessary • Interventions will depend on cause (acute management of delirium if physical cause) • May include use of PRN sedative medication or pharmacological management of acute behavioural disturbance (specialist intervention) • Consider compulsory admission
Special considerations	• Risks of pharmacological management include increased agitation, over sedation, airway compromise and LOC, respiratory and cardiovascular collapse

Musculoskeletal

2WW – Sarcomas – NICE Guidelines[25]

• Bone sarcoma in adults:
  • Consider 2WW referral of adults if an x-ray suggests the possibility of bone sarcoma
• Bone sarcoma in children and young people:
  • Consider a very urgent (within 48h) referral for specialist assessment for children and young people if an x-ray suggests the possibility of bone sarcoma
  • Consider a very urgent direct access x-ray (to be performed within 48h) to assess for bone sarcoma in children and young people with unexplained bone swelling or pain
• Soft tissue sarcoma in adults:
  • Consider an urgent direct access ultrasound scan (to be performed within 2 weeks) to assess for soft tissue sarcoma in adults with an unexplained lump that is increasing in size
  • Consider a suspected cancer pathway referral (for an appointment within 2 weeks) for adults if they have ultrasound scan findings that are suggestive of soft tissue sarcoma or if ultrasound findings are uncertain and clinical concern persists
• Soft tissue sarcoma in children and young people:
  • Consider a very urgent direct access ultrasound scan (to be performed within 48h) to assess for soft tissue sarcoma in children and young people with an unexplained lump that is increasing in size
  • Consider a very urgent referral (for an appointment within 48h) for children and young people if they have ultrasound scan findings that are suggestive of soft tissue sarcoma or if ultrasound findings are uncertain and clinical concern persists

Mechanical Low Back Pain

Classic history	• Consider:
	  • Nature and site
	  • Duration
	  • Radicular symptoms and signs
	  • Psychosocial risk factors
	• Red flags: NICE guidance describes the following red flags[26]:
	  • Cauda equina syndrome:
	    • Severe or progressive bilateral neurological deficit of the legs, such as major motor weakness with knee extension, ankle eversion, or foot dorsiflexion
	    • Recent-onset urinary retention (caused by bladder distension because the sensation of fullness is lost) and/or urinary incontinence (caused by loss of sensation when passing urine)

Mechanical Low Back Pain – cont'd

- Recent-onset faecal incontinence (due to loss of sensation of rectal fullness)
- Perianal or perineal sensory loss (saddle anaesthesia or paraesthesia)
- Unexpected laxity of the anal sphincter
- Spinal fracture:
  - Sudden onset of severe central spinal pain which is relieved by lying down
  - A history of major trauma (such as a road traffic collision or fall from a height), minor trauma, or even just strenuous lifting in people with osteoporosis or those who use corticosteroid
  - Structural deformity of the spine (such as a step from one vertebra to an adjacent vertebra) may be present
  - There may be point tenderness over a vertebral body
- Cancer:
  - Age 50 years of age or more
  - Gradual onset of symptoms
  - Severe unremitting pain that remains when the person is supine, aching night pain that prevents or disturbs sleep, pain aggravated by straining (e.g., at stool, or when coughing or sneezing), and thoracic pain
  - Localised spinal tenderness
  - No symptomatic improvement after 4 to 6 weeks of conservative low back pain therapy
  - Unexplained weight loss
  - Past history of cancer (breast, lung, gastrointestinal, prostate, renal, and thyroid cancers are more likely to metastasise to the spine)
- Infection (such as discitis, vertebral osteomyelitis or spinal epidural abscess):
  - Fever
  - Tuberculosis, or recent urinary tract infection
  - Diabetes
  - History of intravenous drug use
- HIV infection, use of immunosuppressants, or the person is otherwise immunocompromised

Examination considerations	• May include:
	• Gait and posture
	• Range of motion
	• Palpation
	• Heel-toe walk, squat and rise
	• Straight leg raise
	• Reflex, motor and sensory testing
	• Neurology
Important differential diagnoses	• Mechanical low back pain including:
	• Lumbar strain
	• Discogenic (degeneration, herniation)
	• Spinal stenosis
	• Spondylolisthesis
	• Inflammatory arthritis
	• Neoplasm
	• Skin including shingles
	• Urological:
	• UTI
	• Renal colic
	• Prostatitis
	• Pyelonephritis

Mechanical Low Back Pain

	• Gastrointestinal including:
	  • IBS
	  • Pancreatitis
	  • Cholecystitis
	  • Ulcer
	• Gynaecological
	  • Endometriosis
	  • Pelvic inflammatory disease
	• Ruptured AAA
	• Fibromyalgia
	  • Psychogenic

UUC interventions and disposal	• For acute simple back pain:
	• Advice – mobility, exercise, expectant resolution, superficial heat
	• Simple analgesia
	• GP/physiotherapy follow-up if enduring or new sinister features
	• Imaging only useful for small subgroup in whom there is suspicion of red flag conditions[27]; if needed, imaging depends on underlying clinical concerns:
	  • Vertebral fracture: x-ray or possibly CT
	  • Malignancy: x-ray and MRI
	  • Infection: x-ray and MRI
	  • Cauda equina syndrome: MRI
	  • Severe neurologic defects: MRI

Olecranon Bursitis

Classic history	• New swelling over olecranon process • May be painless • May be provoked by low-grade trauma/activity • If hot, tender, localised redness, then consider septic bursitis
Important differential diagnoses	• Simple bursitis • Septic bursitis • Gout • Rheumatoid arthritis

UUC interventions and disposal	• Simple bursitis:
	  • Rest, immobilise
	  • Ice
	  • Analgesia
	• Septic bursitis:
	  • Consider drainage
	  • Antibiotics

Neurology

2WW – Brain and CNS – NICE Guidelines[28]

• Brain and CNS cancer (adults):
  • Consider urgent access (2 week) MRI scan of the brain (or CT scan if MRI is contraindicated) if progressive, sub-acute loss of central neurological function
• Brain and CNS cancer (young people):
  • Consider a very urgent (within 48 h) appointment if newly abnormal cerebellar or other central neurological function

Acute Confusional State/Delirium

Important differential diagnoses	• Infection: any source, worse in elderly • Medication: prescribed, abuse, withdrawal • Neurological: head injury, CVA, subarachnoid, meningitis • Endocrine: Addison, diabetes, thyrotoxicosis, myxoedema • Cardiac – myocardial infarction, failure, endocarditis • Metabolic: hypoxia, hypoglycaemia, hyponatraemia, hypercalcaemia, acidosis, hypercapnia • Psychiatric: depression, dementia, psychosis

History and characteristics	• Predisposing factors:
	  • Comorbidities:
	    ◦ Alcoholism
	    ◦ Chronic pain
	    ◦ Background lung, liver, kidney, heart or brain disease
	    ◦ Terminal illness
	  • Demographic factors:
	    ◦ Older than 65 years
	    ◦ Male
	  • 'Geriatric syndrome':
	    ◦ Dementia
	    ◦ Depression
	    ◦ Elder abuse
	    ◦ Falls
	    ◦ History of delirium
	    ◦ Malnutrition
	    ◦ Polypharmacy
	    ◦ Pressure ulcers
	  • Premorbid state:
	    ◦ Inactivity
	    ◦ Poor functional status
	    ◦ Social isolation
	  • Precipitating factors
	    ◦ Acute insults
	    ◦ Dehydration
	    ◦ Fracture
	    ◦ Infection
	    ◦ Ischaemia – cerebral, cardiac
	    ◦ Medications
	    ◦ Metabolic derangements
	    ◦ Poor nutrition
	    ◦ Severe illness
	    ◦ Shock
	    ◦ Surgery
	    ◦ Controlled pain
	    ◦ Sleep deprivation

Examination considerations	• Full physical • Full mental state
UUC investigations	• FBC • U&E • Glucose • Urinalysis • ECG • CXR
Special considerations	• Consider need for LP, CT, blood cultures

First Fit

Classic history	• Seizure • Tongue biting • Incontinence • Post-ictal state • Check stimulus: alcohol/drug use and withdrawal, hypoglycaemia, arrhythmia, head injury, subarachnoid, CVA/TIA, infection, meningitis, metabolic change
Classic findings	• May be none or post-ictal including drowsiness • Todd Paresis: focal deficit or hemiparesis
Important differential diagnoses	• Syncope • Hyperventilation • Stokes-Adams attacks • Night terrors • Narcolepsy • Rigors • Vertigo • Involuntary movements such as chorea • Hypoglycaemia

UUC investigations	• BM
	• FBC
	• U&E
	• Glucose
	• ECG
	• CXR
	• Blood cultures (if pyrexia)
	• Pregnancy test
	• Possible blood gases, lactate
	• Higher level – NICE recommends following additional investigations for a first seizure[29]:
	  • LP (if encephalitis or subarachnoid haemorrhage is suspected) and drug screening (depending on clinical circumstances)
	  • Early standard electroencephalography, if possible within 24 h
	  • Sleep-deprived electroencephalography within 1 week
	  • High-resolution magnetic resonance imaging, if possible

UUC interventions and disposal	• Emergency CT if: focal signs, head injury, HIV, suspect meningitis/encephalitis, bleeding disorder, on anticoagulants, no resolution of conscious levels • Discharge home with supervision for GP f/u if normal examination and investigations • Admit if >1 seizure or abnormal findings/investigations • Document advice redriving/machinery/swimming/bathing
Special considerations	• DVLA advice

Headache

Important differential diagnoses	• Simple, cluster, tension headaches • Migraine • Benign exertion headache • Minor/viral headache • Head injury • Depression • Dental • Vascular (CVA, subarachnoid, intra-cranial haematoma, AV malformation) • Infection (meningitis, encephalitis) • Trigeminal neuralgia • Drugs (opiate withdrawal) • Inflammatory (GCA)
History and characteristics	• Location, duration, timings – especially 'sudden onset, worst ever' • Relationship with exertion • Visual changes • Altered neurology • Rash • Tenderness
Examination considerations	• Full neurological/cranial nerves (Fig. 7.45) • Fundoscopy
Potential investigations	• FBC • CRP • U&E • Glucose

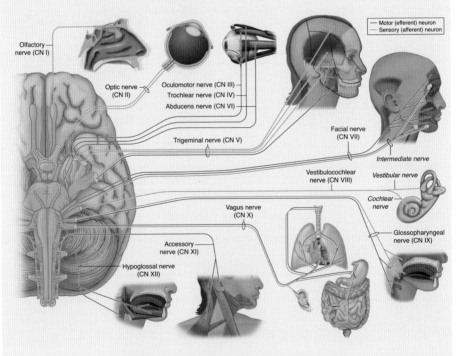

Fig. 7.45 Cranial nerves. (From Patton, 2019.)

Headache

Special considerations	• Current NICE Guidance[30]:
	  • Adults:
	    • Consider an urgent direct access MRI scan of the brain (or CT scan if MRI is contraindicated) (to be performed within 2 weeks) to assess for brain or central nervous system cancer in adults with progressive, sub-acute loss of central neurological function
	  • Children and young people
	    • Consider a very urgent referral (for an appointment within 48 h) for suspected brain or central nervous system cancer in children and young people with newly abnormal cerebellar or other central neurological function
	• Refer urgently if:
	  • 'Thunderclap' headache
	  • Worsening headache with fever
	  • Headache with new neurological, cognitive or personality change
	  • Headache with recent (within 3/12) trauma
	  • Headache triggered by cough, sneeze, Valsalva, exercise
	  • Headache changes with posture
	  • Possible GCA
	  • Possible glaucoma (headache with painful red eye and misty vision)
	  • Substantial change in characteristics of headache
	  • Headache with significant other pathology – HIV, immunosuppression, history malignant

Migraine

Classic history	• Prodrome – blurred vision, visual zigzags, etc. malaise, nausea • Throbbing headache with nausea, sensitivity to noise, light and smell – just want to lie in darkened room • Rare mild unilateral weakness/neurological deficits
Important differential diagnoses	• Subarachnoid haemorrhage • Cluster, simple, tension headache • Giant cell arteritis • Sinusitis • Epilepsy • Trigeminal neuralgia • Space-occupying lesion • Malignant hypertension • Drug (analgesia) related • CO poisoning
UUC interventions and disposal	• Combination therapy: oral triptan and NSAID • Young people 12–17 years: nasal triptan • Antiemetic: metoclopramide or stemetil • Avoid codeine/DHC • Admit if new neurological signs, altered mental state, uncertain diagnosis

Special considerations	• Diagnostic criteria for migraine include[31]:
	  • Repeated attacks of headache lasting 4–72 h that have the following features:
	    • Normal physical examination
	    • No other cause for the headache
	    • At least two of the following features:
	      • Site of pain unilateral
	      • Nature of pain throbbing
	      • Movements aggravates pain
	      • Moderate or severe intensity of pain

Stroke/CVA

Classic history	• Sudden onset motor or sensory loss (lasts >24 h for definition) • 'FAST' positive • Multiple including loss of power/movement or sensation in arm or leg, problems speaking, facial droop, visual loss, expressive or receptive dysphasia
Classic findings	• As above

Relevant anatomy	• Two brain blood supplies:
	  • Internal carotid arteries:
	    ◦ Supplies anterior and middle cerebral arteries
	    ◦ Unilateral weakness/sensory loss, dysphasia, homonymous hemianopia, amaurosis fugax
	  • Basilar arteries:
	    ◦ Supplies posterior cerebral artery
	    ◦ Blackouts, bilateral motor or sensory loss, vertigo, ataxia
	  • Then: anterior and posterior communicating arteries in the Circle of Willis provide collateral circulation in cases of carotid artery stenosis

Important differential diagnoses	• TIA • Hypoglycaemia • Migraine • Meningitis, encephalitis • Brain abscess • Bell palsy • Head injury • Space occupying lesion • Meningitis • Chronic subdural haematoma • Extradural haematoma • Hypertensive encephalopathy • Demyelinating disease, e.g. multiple sclerosis
UUC investigations	• BM • FBC • CRP • U&E • Glucose • ECG • CXR

UUC interventions and disposal	• Correct reversible causes
	• Oxygen
	• DO NOT give aspirin unless intracranial haemorrhage excluded
	• Needs emergency CT if:
	  • Recent onset (possibly 4 h) as may consider thrombolysis
	  • On anticoagulant
	  • Known bleeding disorder
	  • GCS <13
	  • Unexplained progressive or fluctuating symptoms
	  • Papilledema, neck stiffness, fever
	  • Severe headache at onset

Special considerations	• Rosier score for stroke recognition[32]:
	  • Asymmetrical facial weakness (1)
	  • Asymmetrical arm weakness (1)
	  • Asymmetrical leg weakness (1)
	  • Speech disturbance (1)
	  • Visual field defect (1)
	  • LOC or syncope (−1)
	  • Seizure (−1)
	  • Stroke UNLIKELY if score 0 or less
	• DVLA advice

Subarachnoid Haemorrhage

Classic history	• Sudden onset – 'worst pain ever/hit on back of head' • Premonitory headaches in up to 50% • Neck pain, photophobia, vomiting • Unilateral eye pain • Possible seizure, syncope, drowsiness, confusion
Classic findings	• Focal motor and sensory changes • Fundal haemorrhages • Neck stiffness • Varying confusion/consciousness • Reactive hypertension • Extensor plantars
Important differential diagnoses	• Severe migraine • Post-coital benign headache • CVA • Meningitis/encephalitis • Head injury • Glaucoma • GCA

Potential investigations	• ECG (ischaemic changes)
	• FBC
	• Clotting
	• U&E
	• CXR (neurogenic pulmonary oedema)
	• Higher level:
	  • CT
	  • Lumbar puncture

Interventions and disposal options	• Oxygen • IV access • Analgesia • Antiemetic • Short active benzodiazepine
Special considerations	• P1 transfer with pre-alert

Transient Ischaemic Attack

Classic history	• Episode of transient focal motor or sensory loss (lasts < guidance emphasises the need for 24 h for definition)
	• 'FAST' positive
	• Causes:
	  • Thrombo-embolic: AF, mitral stenosis, artificial valves, post-MI, carotid artery stenosis
	  • Hypertension
	  • Polycythaemia/anaemia
	  • Vasculitis: GCA, SLE, polyarteritis nodosa
	  • Sickle cell
	  • Hypoglycaemia
	  • Hypo-perfusion: including arrhythmia, shock
	  • Syphilis

Classic findings	• Resolving neurological deficit • Sources of emboli: arrhythmia (AF), murmurs, bruits

Transient Ischaemic Attack – cont'd

Relevant anatomy	• Two brain blood supplies:
	  • Internal carotid arteries:
	    ◦ Supplies anterior and middle cerebral arteries
	    ◦ Unilateral weakness/sensory loss, dysphasia, homonymous hemianopia, amaurosis fugax
	  • Basilar arteries:
	    ◦ Supplies posterior cerebral artery
	    ◦ Blackouts, bilateral motor or sensory loss, vertigo, ataxia
	  • Then: anterior and posterior communicating arteries in the 'Circle of Willis' provide collateral circulation in cases of carotid artery stenosis

Important differential diagnoses	• Hypoglycaemia
	• Migraine
	• Meningitis, encephalitis
	• Brain abscess
	• Bell palsy
	• Head injury
	• Space-occupying lesion
	• Epilepsy:
	• Structural brain lesions:
	  • Tumours
	  • Chronic subdural haematomas
	  • Vascular malformation
	• Other non-vascular causes:
	  • Multiple sclerosis
	  • Meniere disease
	  • Hypoglycaemia
	  • Hysteria
	• In patients with transient monocular symptoms:
	  • Giant cell arteritis
	  • Malignant hypertension
	  • Glaucoma
	  • Papilledema
	• Transient global amnesia

UUC investigations	• BM
	• FBC
	• CRP
	• U&E
	• Glucose
	• ECG
	• CXR
	• Higher level:
	  • Echo
	  • Carotid duplex scanning
	  • CT

UUC interventions and disposal	• Correct reversible causes
	• Oxygen if required
	• ABCD2
	• NICE guidance emphasises the need for review within 24h of a patient with a TIA[33]:
	  • Offer aspirin (300mg daily), unless contraindicated, to people who have had a suspected TIA, to be started immediately
	  • Refer immediately people who have had a suspected TIA for specialist assessment and investigation, to be seen within 24h of onset of symptoms

Transient Ischaemic Attack

	• Do **not** use scoring systems, such as ABCD2, to assess risk of subsequent stroke or to inform urgency of referral for people who have had a suspected or confirmed TIA
	• Offer secondary prevention, in addition to aspirin, as soon as possible after the diagnosis of TIA is confirmed
	• Admit if >1 TIA in past week or continuing symptoms or residual defect (i.e. therefore not a TIA)
Special considerations	• DVLA advice

Obstetrics and Gynaecology

2WW – Gynaecological – NICE Guidelines[34]

- Ovarian cancer (apply to women aged 18 and over):
  - Refer urgently if physical examination identifies ascites and/or a pelvic or abdominal mass (which is not obviously uterine fibroids)
  - Carry out appropriate tests in primary care if a woman (especially if 50 or over) reports having any of the following symptoms on a persistent or frequent basis – particularly more than 12 times per month:
    - Persistent abdominal distension (women often refer to this as 'bloating')
    - Feeling full (early satiety) and/or loss of appetite
    - Pelvic or abdominal pain
    - Increased urinary urgency and/or frequency
  - Consider carrying out appropriate tests in primary care if a woman reports unexplained weight loss, fatigue or changes in bowel habit
  - Advise any woman who is not suspected of having ovarian cancer to return to her GP if her symptoms become more frequent and/or persistent
  - Carry out appropriate tests for ovarian cancer in any woman of 50 or over who has experienced symptoms within the last 12 months that suggest irritable bowel syndrome (IBS), because IBS rarely presents for the first time in women of this age
  - Measure serum CA125 in primary care in women with symptoms that suggest ovarian cancer
  - If serum CA125 is 35 IU/mL or greater, arrange an ultrasound scan of the abdomen and pelvis
  - If the ultrasound suggests ovarian cancer, refer the woman urgently for further investigation
  - For any woman who has normal serum CA125 (less than 35 IU/mL), or CA125 of 35 IU/mL or greater but a normal ultrasound:
    - Assess her carefully for other clinical causes of her symptoms and investigate if appropriate
    - If no other clinical cause is apparent, advise her to return to her GP if her symptoms become more frequent and/or persistent
- Endometrial cancer:
  - 2WW referral if aged 55 and over with post-menopausal bleeding (unexplained vaginal bleeding more than 12 months after menstruation has stopped because of the menopause)
  - Consider a suspected cancer pathway referral (for an appointment within 2 weeks) for endometrial cancer in women aged under 55 with post-menopausal bleeding
  - Consider a direct access ultrasound scan to assess for endometrial cancer in women aged 55 and over with:
    - Unexplained symptoms of vaginal discharge who:
      - Are presenting with these symptoms for the first time or
      - Have thrombocytosis or
      - Report haematuria, or
    - Visible haematuria and:
      - Low haemoglobin levels or
      - Thrombocytosis or
      - High blood glucose levels
- Cervical cancer:
  - Consider 2WW referral if, on examination, the appearance of their cervix is consistent with cervical cancer
- Vulval cancer:
  - Consider 2WW referral of women with an unexplained vulval lump, ulceration or bleeding
- Vaginal cancer:
  - Consider 2WW referral of women with an unexplained palpable mass in or at the entrance to the vagina

Abnormal Vaginal Bleeding

Important differential diagnoses	• Dysfunctional uterine bleeding • Hormonal (including iatrogenic) • Fibroids • Endometriosis • Pelvic inflammatory disease • IUCD • Polyp • Carcinoma • Hypothyroidism • Retained tampon (must be considered and excluded) • Cervical erosion/ectropion • Pregnancy related

UUC investigations and disposal	• Dependant on presenting history, may involve:
	  • FBC
	  • Swabs
	  • GP follow-up

Special considerations	• If appropriate treat for shock

Ectopic Pregnancy

Classic history	• Consider in any round woman presenting with abdominal pain or vaginal bleeding
	• Sudden severe lower abdominal pain
	• Radiation to shoulder if diaphragmatic irritation
	• D&V
	• Collapse
	• Vaginal bleeding
	• General pregnancy symptoms
	• Risk factors:
	  • Pelvic inflammatory disease
	  • Adhesions
	  • Previous ectopic
	  • Endometriosis
	  • Assisted conception
	  • IUCD
	  • POP
	  • Congenital abnormalities
	  • Ovarian/uterine tumours

Classic findings	• 'Acute abdomen' • Shock • Pelvic tenderness • Adnexal tenderness • Abdominal distension
Important differential diagnoses	• See Acute Abdominal Pain table • See Gynaecological Pain table
UUC investigations	• Pregnancy test • USS (check intrauterine pregnancy)
UUC interventions and disposal	• Oxygen • Large bore cannula • IV fluids • Analgesia • P1 transfer with pre-alert
Special considerations	• Commonest cause of maternal mortality in first trimester

Gynaecological Pain

Important differential diagnoses	• See Acute Abdominal Pain table
	• Gynaecological causes:
	  • Ectopic pregnancy
	  • Threatened abortion
	  • Physiological dysmenorrhea
	  • Endometriosis
	  • Rupture corpus luteum
	  • Mittelschmerz
	  • Uterine perforation
	  • Fibroids
	  • Ovarian torsion
	  • Ovarian cyst
	  • Pelvic inflammatory disease

History and characteristics	• Sudden onset (ovarian torsion, vascular event) • Insidious, chronic (infection, inflammation) • Radiation to back or legs • Vaginal discharge • Vaginal bleeding • Date or missed LMP • Relationship to menstrual cycle • Check pre-, peri- or post-menopausal

Menorrhagia

Classic history	• Various descriptions of excessive menstrual loss:
	  • Unusual for the woman
	  • Subjectively excessive
	  • Interfering with normal quality of life
	  • Objectively involving >80 mL loss
	  • Associated with flooding, clots, use of towels rather than tampons
	  • Associated with excessive pain
	• Ask about:
	  • Previous cycle history including regularity
	  • Post-coital bleeding
	  • Intermenstrual bleeding
	  • Discharge
	  • Smear history
	  • Separate bleeding/bruising

Classic findings Important differential diagnosis	• Consider anaemia • Idiopathic • Dysfunctional uterine bleeding • Hormone imbalance • Fibroids and polyps • Cancer • Polyps • Pregnancy-related • Bleeding disorders • Medication (including anticoagulants, hormonal) • Thyroid disorders • Liver or kidney disease

Menorrhagia – cont'd

UUC investigations	• If relevant:
	  • FBC
	  • Clotting
	  • U&E
	  • LFT
	  • Higher level:
	    • Ferritin
	    • Female hormones
	    • TFTs
	• Depending on associated features and background concerns may need:
	  • Physical examination:
	    • NICE recommend examine if[35]:
	      • History of menorrhagia plus other related symptoms (persistent intermenstrual bleeding, pelvic pain and/or pressure symptoms, which might suggest uterine cavity abnormality, histological abnormality, adenomyosis or fibroid)
	      • Before investigations are conducted
	  • Smear
	  • Swabs
	  • Ultrasound

UUC interventions and disposal	• Short course medical treatment suitable for UUC delivery includes:
	  • Tranexamic acid
	  • NSAIDs
	• Other treatments available via GP include levonorgestrel-releasing IUS, oral contraceptives, referral for consideration of surgical options

Special considerations	• Biopsy would be indicated if:
	  • Persistent intermenstrual bleeding, and, in women aged 45 and over, treatment failure or ineffective treatment
	• USS if:
	  • Uterus is palpable abdominally
	  • Vaginal examination reveals a pelvic mass of uncertain origin
	  • Failure of pharmaceutical treatment
	• Hysteroscopy if USS inconclusive, e.g., to determine the exact location of a fibroid or the exact nature of abnormality
	• Refer urgently if physical examination identifies ascites and/or a pelvic or abdominal mass
	• Refer using 2WW pathway if pelvic mass associated with any other features of cancer (such as unexplained bleeding or weight loss)
	• Refer routinely if:
	  • Complications such as compressive symptoms from large fibroids (e.g. dyspareunia, pelvic pain or discomfort, constipation or urinary symptoms)
	  • Iron deficiency anaemia which has failed to respond to treatment
	  • Menorrhagia has not improved despite initial treatment

Pre-Eclampsia

Classic history	• Requires two or more of:
	  • Hypertension >140/90
	  • Proteinuria
	  • Oedema
	• Classic symptoms:
	  • Confusion, headache, tremor, twitching, abdominal pain, visual disturbance, swelling, fits
	• Risk factors:
	  • Age ≥40
	  • Nulliparity
	  • Last pregnancy >10 years ago
	  • personal, family history of pre-eclampsia
	  • BMI ≥30
	  • Pre-existing hypertension, vascular disease, renal disease
	  • Multiple pregnancy

Important differential diagnoses	• Hypertension • Renal failure
UUC investigations	• FBC • U&E • LFT • Clotting • BM • ECG • Foetal doppler

UUC interventions and disposal	• Start antihypertensives (typically labetalol) if BP >140/90 mm Hg but no other concerns
	• Needs GP/midwife f/u including twice weekly FBC, LFT, U&E, BP monitoring, foetal monitoring
	• Admit if:
	  • BP 140/90 – 159/109 mm Hg and there are clinical concerns for mother or baby
	  • BP >160/110 mm Hg

Special considerations	• Target BP once treated is ≤135/85 mm Hg
	• HELLP syndrome:
	  • Haemolysis
	  • Elevated
	  • LFTs
	  • Low platelets

Vaginal Bleeding in Pregnancy

Important differential diagnoses (pregnancy-related)	• Spontaneous abortion • Ectopic • Trophoblastic disease • Placental abruption • Placenta praevia

Special considerations	• If appropriate treat for shock:
	  • Oxygen
	  • Large bore cannula
	  • IV fluids
	  • FBC, clotting
	  • P1 transfer, pre-alert
	• Anti-D:
	  • Follow guidelines if possible foetomaternal bleeding in a rhesus-negative mother

Vaginal Discharge

Important differential diagnoses	• Physiological
	• General gynaecological:
	  • Atrophic vaginitis
	  • Cervical and endometrial carcinoma
	  • Fistulae
	  • Foreign body including retained tampon (also consider toxic shock syndrome)
	  • Polyp
	  • Pregnancy
	• Infections:
	  • Thrush
	  • General bacterial
	  • Chlamydia
	  • Trichomonas
	  • Parasites

History and characteristics	• Normal vs changes • Timing (including relation to cycle) • Tenderness • Nature • Pruritus • Odour • Superficial dyspareunia • Sexual history • Dysuria • Abnormal bleeding (PCB, IMB)

UUC investigations	• High vaginal swab MC&S
	• Higher level:
	  • STI testing
	  • GP follow-up

Ophthalmology

Blepharitis

Classic history	• Usually bilateral • Red irritated eyelids • Eye discomfort, burning, itching • Mild photophobia • Blurred vision • Potential atopy/sensitivity history
Classic findings	• Red, inflamed eyelid margins • Crusting • Conjunctival hyperaemia

UUC interventions and disposal	• Advice:
	  • Remove irritants including makeup
	  • Regular cleaning and massage with warm facecloth
	• Antibiotics:
	  • Topical or oral
	• Under expert advice:
	  • Short course topical corticosteroids

Conjunctivitis

Classic history	• Gritty, irritated eyes • Purulent (yellow sticky) or watery discharge • Photophobia • Blurred vision • Exposure to irritants
Classic findings	• Red, irritated eyes • Hyperaemic conjunctivae
Important differential diagnoses	• Acute iritis • Glaucoma • Blepharitis

UUC interventions and disposal	• Advice, expect resolution in most
	• Broad spectrum topical antibiotic:
	  • Definitely beneficial if positive MC&S
	  • Possibly beneficial:
	    • Improves early (days 2–5) clinical remission with NNT of 7
	    • Improves early microbiological remission with NNT of 3

Special considerations	• Refer to ophthalmology if:
	  • Neonatal conjunctivitis
	  • Chronic conjunctivitis
	  • No response to treatment after 7 days
	  • Associated corneal changes
	  • Blurring of vision or pain
	  • Dry eye syndromes

Corneal Abrasion and Ulcers

Classic history	• Trauma/FB • Pain • Watery eyes • Photophobia • Blepharospasm
Important differential diagnoses	• Conjunctivitis • Corneal ulcer
UUC investigations	• Fluorescein staining • Thorough examination including eyelid eversion
UUC interventions and disposal	• Topical antibiotics • Eye padding • Analgesia
Special considerations	• Corneal ulcer is an ophthalmic emergency

Peri-Orbital Cellulitis

Classic history	• Pain, redness and swelling around eye • Possible local infection

Classic findings	• Need to distinguish between pre-septal and orbital cellulitis with low threshold/degree of suspicion as delayed recognition of the signs and symptoms of orbital cellulitis can lead to serious complications
	• Pre-septal cellulitis:
	  • Acute onset of swelling, redness, warmth and eyelid tenderness
	  • Eyelid oedema in the absence of orbital signs such as gaze restriction and proptosis
	  • Fever, malaise, irritability in children
	  • Ptosis
	• Orbital cellulitis
	  • Anterior features:
	    • Acute onset of unilateral swelling of conjunctiva and lids
	    • Oedema, erythema, pain, chemosis
	  • Orbital features:
	    • External eye muscle ophthalmoplegia and proptosis
	    • Decreased visual acuity and chemosis
	    • Proptosis
	    • Pain with movement of the eye
	    • Restriction of eye movements
	    • Blurred vision, reduced visual acuity
	    • Diplopia
	• Features which should increase the suspicion of orbital cellulitis include:
	  • Decreased visual acuity, proptosis and external ophthalmoplegia
	  • Temperature >37.5°C and leucocytosis resulting in fever (especially in children)

Relevant anatomy	• Extension of infection from nasal sinuses or nearby skin
	• Sometimes spread from distant site in children
	• Orbital septum:
	  • Membranous sheet which acts as the anterior boundary of the orbit
	  • Arises from the periosteum around the orbital margin
	  • Centrally, it fuses into the tarsal plates
	  • Separates the eyelids from the contents of the orbital cavity
	  • Provides a barrier against spread of infection between the pre-septal space anteriorly to post-septal space

Important differential diagnosis	• Chalazion • Allergy • Angio-oedema • Thyroid eye disease • Orbital tumours • Insect bites • Graves disease • Rhabdomyosarcoma • Pseudo-tumour

Peri-Orbital Cellulitis

UUC investigations	• FBC
	• Inflammatory and sepsis markers
	• Higher:
	  • CT
	  • MRI

UUC interventions and disposal	• Low grade concerns:
	  • First choice antibiotics: co-amoxiclav + metronidazole if anaerobes suspected
	  • Alternative: clarithromycin
	  • Hot compresses
	  • Nasal decongestants
	• Emergency referral to secondary care if:
	  • All children with suspected pre-septal cellulitis
	  • All patients with suspected orbital cellulitis
	  • All patients with features of either condition who are systemically unwell
	  • All patients in whom there is doubt over the diagnosis
	  • Any patient not responding to treatment for pre-septal cellulitis
	  • When drainage of a lid abscess is required.
	• Consider discussing with specialist as true peri-orbital cellulitis requires:
	  • Urgent referral
	  • Immediate IV antibiotics
	  • Cultures
	  • Surgical drainage indicated in suppurative pre-septal cellulitis

Special considerations	• Most often haemophilus influenzae, streptococcus pneumoniae and staphylococci
	• Complications can include:
	  • Cavernous sinus thrombosis
	  • Erosion of orbital bones
	  • Brain abscess
	  • Meningitis

The Red Eye

Important differential diagnoses	• Conjunctivitis • Foreign body • Penetrating eye injury • Iritis • Acute glaucoma • Herpes • Allergy • Episcleritis • Scleritis • Corneal abrasion • Corneal ulceration • Keratitis

The Red Eye – cont'd

Special considerations	• Refer ophthalmology if:
	• Loss of visual acuity
	• Abnormal pupillary reactions
	• Conjunctival injection is most marked around the pupil (keratitis, corneal ulcer or intraocular pathology)
	• Corneal ulceration
	• Possible penetrating injury
	• Cloudy fundus
	• No improvement after topical treatment

Respiratory

2WW – Lung – NICE Guidelines[36]

- Lung cancer:
  - 2WW referral for patients who:
    - Have chest x-ray findings that suggest lung cancer or
    - Are aged 40 and over with unexplained haemoptysis
  - Offer an urgent CXR (within 2 weeks) to people aged 40 and over if they have 2 or more of the following unexplained symptoms, or if they have ever smoked and have 1 or more of the following unexplained symptoms:
    - Cough
    - Fatigue
    - Shortness of breath
    - Chest pain
    - Weight loss
    - Appetite loss
  - Consider an urgent CXR (within 2 weeks) to people aged 40 and over with any of the following:
    - Persistent or recurrent chest infection
    - Finger clubbing
    - Supraclavicular lymphadenopathy or persistent cervical lymphadenopathy
    - Chest signs consistent with lung cancer
    - Thrombocytosis
- Mesothelioma:
  - 2WW referral if CXR findings suggest mesothelioma
  - Offer urgent CXR (within 2 weeks) to people aged 40 and over, if:
    - They have 2 or more of the following unexplained symptoms, or
    - They have 1 or more of the following unexplained symptoms and have ever smoked, or
    - They have 1 or more of the following unexplained symptoms and have been exposed to asbestos:
      - Cough
      - Fatigue
      - Shortness of breath
      - Chest pain
      - Weight loss
      - Appetite loss
  - Consider urgent CXR (within 2 weeks) for people aged 40 and over with either:
    - Finger clubbing or
    - Chest signs compatible with pleural disease

Acute Asthma – Moderate

Classic history	• Wheeze • SOB • Chest tightness • Cough • Triggers: cold, exercise, allergens, irritants • Variation: worse night and early morning
Classic findings	• Wheeze • Peak flow 50%–75% of predicted
Important differential diagnoses	• Varies with age • URTI • Nasal congestion and post-nasal drip • GORD • Bronchiectasis • Primary ciliary dyskinesia • Cystic fibrosis – excessive cough and mucus production, gastrointestinal symptoms • Vocal cord dysfunction – dyspnoea, inspiratory wheezing (stridor) • Hyperventilation: anxiety, pain, panic • COPD

Potential investigations	• PEFR
	• CXR
	• Infection markers
	• Higher level:
	  • FENO
	  • Spirometry

Interventions and disposal options	• Depends on severity (also see severe/life threatening table) • Nebulised then inhaled B-agonist • Nebulised ipratropium bromide • Steroid (prednisolone) • Antibiotics for infective exacerbations
Special considerations	• Review inhaler technique • Follow-up with GP within 2 days • Safety net/worsening advice

Refer to BTS Council guidelines at https://www.brit-thoracic.org.uk/quality-improvement/guidelines/asthma/.

Acute Asthma – Life-Threatening

Classic history	• Wheeze • SOB • Cannot complete sentence • Exhaustion, confusion, coma, fearful

Classic findings	• By definition, any 1 from:
	  • Cyanosis
	  • Exhaustion, confusion, coma
	  • Feeble respiratory effort
	  • SpO_2 <92%
	  • Silent chest
	  • Bradycardia, arrythmia, hypotension
	  • pO_2 <8kPa
	  • Normal cCO_2 (4.6–6.0kPa)
	  • Peak flow <33% best or predicted

Acute Asthma – Life-Threatening – cont'd

Potential investigations	• PEFR • CXR • ABG • Infection markers
Interventions and disposal options	• High flow oxygen • Sit patient up • ABC, exclude pneumothorax • Cannulate • High-dose nebulised B-agonist • Nebulised ipratropium bromide • Steroid (prednisolone oral or hydrocortisone IV) • Consider IV fluids • P1 transfer • Pre-alert

Refer to BTS Council guidelines at https://www.brit-thoracic.org.uk/quality-improvement/guidelines/asthma/.

COPD – Exacerbation

Classic history	• SOB • Productive cough • Wheeze
Classic findings	• Acute worsening of respiratory symptoms • Dyspnoea • Tachypnoea • Cough • Sputum production • Accessory muscles • Lip pursing • Hyperinflation • Wheeze/tight chest • Coarse crepe • Cyanosis • Plethora • Associated: fatigue, weight loss
Important differential diagnoses	• Asthma • Pulmonary oedema • Pneumothorax • PE • LRTI • Malignancy • TB

Potential investigations	• CXR
	• ABG
	• FBC
	• U&E
	• Glucose
	• CRP
	• Lactate
	• ECG (tall P waves, RBBB, RHV)
	• Sputum MC&S
	• Higher level:
	  • Spirometry
	  • CT thorax

COPD – Exacerbation

| Interventions and disposal options | • Moderate:
  • Nebulised B-agonist
  • Nebulised ipratropium bromide
  • Steroid (prednisolone oral or hydrocortisone IV)
  • Oral antibiotics
• Severe:
  • Oxygen (aim for SpO_2 88%–92%)
  • Sit patient up
  • ABC, exclude pneumothorax
  • Cannulate
  • High dose nebulised B-agonist
  • Nebulised ipratropium bromide
  • Steroid (prednisolone oral or hydrocortisone IV)
  • Consider IV fluids
  • IV Antibiotics
  • P1 transfer
  • Pre-alert
• Indications for admission include:
  • Acute respiratory failure
  • Worsening SOB/confusion
  • New oedema or cyanosis
  • Significant co-morbidities
  • Failure to respond to treatment
  • Lack of support |

Refer to BTS Council guidelines at https://www.brit-thoracic.org.uk/quality-improvement/guidelines/copd/.

Croup

Classic history	• 6 months to 3 years (can be older) • Barking cough • Prodromal URTI • Fever • Fast breathing
Important differential diagnoses	• Epiglottitis (if suspected DO NOT EXAMINE THROAT) • Tracheitis • Tonsilitis/peri-tonsillar abscess • Foreign body • Angioedema • Asthma • URTI/LRTI

Interventions and disposal options	• Steroids:
	  • Single dose oral dexamethasone, 0.15 mg/kg body weight, or
	  • Oral prednisolone 1–2 mg/kg body weight
	• Repeat 24 h later
	• Antipyretics
	• Avoid antibiotics
	• Steam no longer recommended
	• Routine ENT referral if recurrent (>2 episodes/year)
	• Admit if:
	  • Moderate to severe symptoms
	  • Immunocompromised
	  • <6 months old
	  • Poor fluid intake

Pleural Effusion

Classic history
- Shortness of breath
- Dull ache
- Most common causes:
  - Infection
  - Lung infarction
  - TB
  - Malignancy
  - Organ failure
  - Consider heart failure

Classic findings
- Stony dull percussion (picks up from 500 mL)
- Tachypnoea
- Bronchial breathing
- Reduced movement (affected side)
- Vocal fremitus

Potential investigations
- FBC, U&E, LFT
- CXR (picks up from 250 mL)
- Higher level:
  - USS
  - CT
  - BNP
  - Transthoracic echo
  - Diagnostic pleural aspiration including cytology

Interventions and disposal options
- Need to identify underlying cause
- Therapeutic aspirations, chest drains may be appropriate

Pneumonia/LRTI

Classic history
- SOB
- Productive cough
- Fever
- Pleuritic chest pain
- Myalgia
- Rigors
- Haemoptysis
- Exhaustion, confusion

Classic findings
- Pyrexia
- Inspiratory crackles
- Consolidation
- Decreased percussion (affected side)
- Pleural rub

Important differential diagnoses
- Pulmonary oedema
- Pulmonary infarction
- Pulmonary vasculitis
- Carcinoma
- Acute pancreatitis
- Sub-phrenic abscess

Potential investigations
- FBC
- CRP
- Lactate
- CXR
- ABG
- Sputum MC&S

Pneumonia/LRTI

Interventions and disposal options	• Mild to moderate (CURB-65 score 0 or 1):
	  • Oral antibiotics
	  • Analgesia
	  • GP follow-up
	• Severe (CURB-65 score ≥3):
	  • IV antibiotics
	  • Fluids
	  • Admit
	  • P1 transfer
	  • Pre-alert

Special considerations	• Always consider SIRS/sepsis (see sepsis table)
	• Consider 'secondary' pneumonia, i.e. related to underlying neoplasm
	• CRB-65[37]:
	  • Score for pneumonia, one point each for:
	    • Confusion
	    • RR ≥ 30/min
	    • Low BP (systolic < 90 mm Hg or diastolic < 60 mm Hg)
	    • Age ≥ 65 years
	  • Risk of death:
	    • 0: Low risk (<1% mortality)
	    • 1 or 2: Medium risk (1%–10% mortality)
	    • 3 or 4: High risk (>10% mortality)
	  • Place of care:
	    • 0: home
	    • 1: use clinical judgement either home or hospital
	    • 2 or more: consider admission
	• NICE guidance suggests use CRP results to guide treatment[38]:
	  • <20: no antibiotics
	  • 20–100: delayed script
	  • >100: Immediate antibiotics

Refer to BTS Council guidelines at https://www.brit-thoracic.org.uk/quality-improvement/guidelines/copd/.

Spontaneous Pneumothorax

Classic history	• Possibly asymptomatic • Sudden SOB • Unilateral pleuritic chest pain
Classic findings	• Dyspnoea • Tachypnoea • Tachycardia • Hyper-resonant to percussion (affected side) • Decreased breath sounds (affected side) • Inspiratory 'click' • Tracheal deviation (late stage)
Relevant anatomy	• Tension decompression site: mid clavicular line, 2nd intercostal space
Important differential diagnoses	• Tension pneumothorax

Potential investigations	• CXR
	• ABG
	• Higher level:
	  • CT
	  • USS

Spontaneous Pneumothorax – cont'd	

Interventions and disposal options	• Tension: decompress
	• Otherwise:
	  • High flow oxygen
	  • Cannulation
	  • Erect CXR
	  • Potential aspiration
	  • Potential drain
	  • Potentially admit

Urogenital

2WW – Urology – NICE Guidelines[39]

- Prostate cancer:
  - 2WW referral if prostate feels malignant on digital rectal examination
  - Consider a prostate-specific antigen (PSA) test and digital rectal examination to assess for prostate cancer in men with:
    - Any lower urinary tract symptoms, such as nocturia, urinary frequency, hesitancy, urgency or retention or
    - Erectile dysfunction or
    - Visible haematuria
  - 2WW referral if PSA levels are above the age-specific reference range
- Bladder cancer:
  - 2WW referral if:
    - Aged 45 and over and have:
      - Unexplained visible haematuria without urinary tract infection or
      - Visible haematuria that persists or recurs after successful treatment of urinary tract infection, or
      - Aged 60 and over and have unexplained non-visible haematuria and either dysuria or a raised white cell count on a blood test
  - Consider non-urgent referral if aged 60 and over with recurrent or persistent unexplained urinary tract infection
- Renal cancer:
  - 2WW referral if aged 45 and over and have:
    - Unexplained visible haematuria without urinary tract infection or
    - Visible haematuria that persists or recurs after successful treatment of urinary tract infection
- Testicular cancer:
  - Consider 2WW referral if non-painful enlargement or change in shape or texture of the testis
  - Consider direct access ultrasound scan for testicular cancer in men with unexplained or persistent testicular symptoms
- Penile cancer:
  - Consider 2WW referral if have either:
    - A penile mass or ulcerated lesion, where a sexually transmitted infection has been excluded as a cause, or
    - A persistent penile lesion after treatment for a sexually transmitted infection has been completed
    - Consider 2WW referral if unexplained or persistent symptoms affecting the foreskin or glans

Acute Epididymitis/Epididymo-Orchitis	

Classic history	• Gradual onset testicular ache
	• Subsequent testicular/epididymal swelling
	• Dysuria
	• Urethral discharge
	• Fever and rigors
	• Predisposing factors:
	  • UTI
	  • STI
	  • Urological procedures

Acute Epididymitis/Epididymo-Orchitis

Classic findings	• Acutely tender epididymis • Testis low in scrotum
Important differential diagnoses	• Torsion • Hydrocele • Varicocele
UUC investigations	• FBC • MSU • Urethral swab • AXR (if calculi) • Higher level: • IVU or USS
UUC interventions and disposal	• Refer if concern retorsion • Antibiotics – typically ciprofloxacin • Analgesia • Scrotal elevation • Rest

Acute Prostatitis

Classic history	• Fever
	• Urgency
	• Peri-anal pain
	• Urethral discharge
	• Haematuria
	• Complications can include:
	  • Retention
	  • Abscess
	  • Pyelonephritis
	  • UTI
	  • Epididymo-orchitis

Classic findings	• PR: tender prostate
UUC investigations	• Urinalysis (protein)
UUC interventions and disposal	• Send urine sample for MC&S • GP follow-up – consider other causes • Admit if severe/complication

Balanitis

Classic history	• Discomfort around/under foreskin and head of penis • Dried, painful, cracking skin • Discharge, sometimes bleeding • Painful intercourse • Pain passing urine • Non-circumcised typically
Classic findings	• As above
Important differential diagnoses	• Cancer head penis • Urethritis/STI • Consider underlying diabetes if recurrent
UUC investigations	• Swab

Balanitis – cont'd

UUC interventions and disposal	• Topical or oral antifungals if suspecting fungal/candida infection • Topical or oral antibiotics if suspecting bacterial infection • May be combined with topical steroid • Refer GUM clinic if ulceration, urethritis, lymphadenopathy • GP follow-up if circumcision being considered (local prior approval criteria)

Renal Colic

Classic history	• Severe 'loin to groin' pain, in waves • Nausea, vomiting, pallor, sweating • Features of UTI • Haematuria • Rarely obstruction/retention • Can spread to testes/penis/labia
Classic findings	• Severe pain, doubled over • Pallor • Sweatiness • Tachycardia • Loin tenderness • Pyrexia/rigors suggests associated infection
Important differential diagnoses	• Leaking aortic aneurysm • Pyelonephritis • Appendicitis • Salpingitis • Drug seeking behaviour • Peritonitis

UUC investigations	• MSU (haematuria)
	• U&E, creatinine, glucose
	• Higher level:
	  • USS/doppler
	  • CT KUB
	  • IVU
	  • Blood: calcium, phosphate, urate

UUC interventions and disposal	• Analgesia – IV opioid, NSAID (diclofenac PR)
	• Antiemetic
	• Do not 'push fluids'
	• GP f/u for confirmatory investigations
	• Admit if:
	  • Pain persists
	  • Obstruction
	  • Infection
	  • Sepsis
	  • Renal impairment
	  • Cannot tolerate oral fluids

Special considerations	• Larger calculi may cause retention

Testicular Torsion

Classic history	• Sudden onset severe unilateral testicular pain and swelling • Abdominal discomfort • Vomiting
Classic findings	• Red, tender, swollen testis • Angell sign – other testicle may lie horizontal • Prehn sign – physical lifting of the testicles relieves the pain of epididymitis but not torsion
Important differential diagnoses	• Acute epididymo-orchitis • Torsion of hydatid of Morgagni • Strangulated inguinal hernia • Testicular trauma
UUC investigations	• None – refer immediately based on clinical suspicion
UUC interventions and disposal	• Analgesia • Urgent surgical referral

Urinary Retention

Classic history	• Inability to pass urine
	• Extreme discomfort
	• Common male causes:
	  • Prostatic hyperplasia/cancer
	  • Urethral stricture
	  • Post-operative
	  • Prostatitis
	  • Drugs
	  • Pain including UTI
	• Common female causes:
	  • Retroverted gravid uterus
	  • Atrophic urethritis
	  • Multiple sclerosis
	• Other general causes:
	  • Urethral stones
	  • Constipation
	  • Pelvic tumour
	  • Genital herpes

Classic findings	• Tender, enlarged bladder dull to precision
Relevant anatomy	• Importance of fitting correct sized (especially male vs female) catheter
UUC investigations	• Bladder scan • FBC, U&E • AXR (if calculi)

UUC interventions and disposal	• Catheterise unless:
	  • Following trauma or as result of urethral stenosis
	  • Previous prostatectomy
	  • Known difficult catheterisation
	• Drain and record urine
	• Urinalysis
	• MC&S
	• F/u GP or urology

Urinary Tract Infection

Classic history	• Lower UTI: • Dysuria, frequency, haematuria, supra-pubic discomfort, urgency, burning, cloudy offensive urine • Upper UTI: • Malaise, fever, loin/back pain, vomiting, riggers
Classic findings	• Dipstick urinalysis: positive for blood, leucocytes, protein, nitrites
Important differential diagnoses	• Pyelonephritis • Vulvo-vaginitis • Thrush • Renal calculi

UUC interventions and disposal	• Female uncomplicated:
	 • Treat if moderate to severe urgency or frequency, positive dipstick for blood, leucocytes AND nitrite or symptoms impairing daily function
	 • Lower UTI: 3- to 6-day oral antibiotics (e.g. nitrofurantoin/trimethoprim)
	 • Upper UTI: ciprofloxacin 500 mh bd 7/7 or co-amoxiclav 625 mg TDS 14/7
	• Elderly with asymptomatic bacteriuria:
	 • No antibiotic treatment unless symptomatic
	• Pregnancy:
	 • Send MC&S
	 • Treat symptomatic and asymptomatic bacteriuria (e.g. with amoxicillin)
	 • 7/7 course
	 • Test MC&S for cure afterwards
	• Men:
	 • Given difficulty in distinguishing from prostatitis, consider 2-week course (ciprofloxacin/trimethoprim/co-amoxiclav)
	 • Needs urology referral if:
	  • Recurrent (>1 episode in 3 months)
	  • Upper UTI
	  • Fail to respond to antibiotics
	• Catheterised:
	 • 7 days (ciprofloxacin or co-amoxiclav)
	• Children:
	 • Refer urgently if:
	  • <3 months with suspected UTI
	  • Any age actually unwell with UTI
	  • >3 months with pyelonephritis but cannot tolerate oral antibiotics

Special considerations	• F/u with GP for onward referral if: • Male • Females with recurrent UTI • Pregnancy • Genito-urinary malformation • Immunosuppression • Renal impairment

Vascular

Acute Limb Ischaemia

Classic history	• Pain • Paraesthesia (then anaesthesia) • Pallor (then mottled, cyanosed) • Pulselessness • Paralysis • Perishing cold • Risk factors: • Embolic: AF, post-MI, prosthetic valves, rheumatic heart disease, diabetes, smoking, hypertension, hypercholesterolaemia
Classic findings	• Above • Embolic: clear demarcation, normal pulses • Thrombotic: chronic vascular insufficiency
UUC interventions and disposal	• Effective analgesia • Correct hypovolaemia • P1 transfer vascular team

Deep Vein Thrombosis

Classic history	• Pain
	• Swelling
	• Warmth
	• Tenderness
	• Risk factors:
	   • Prolonged immobility
	   • Post-surgery
	   • Malignancy
	   • IV drug use
	   • Previous DVT/PE
	   • Thrombophilia
	   • Recent Covid 19 infection

Classic findings	• Swelling (calf >3 cm)
	• Warmth
	• Tenderness
	• Predisposing factors:
	   • Recent immobility/paralysis
	   • Recent major surgery
	   • Pregnancy/postpartum
	   • Malignancy and chemotherapy
	   • Oral contraceptive therapy
	   • Previous venous thromboembolism
	   • Thrombophilia
	   • Bed rest longer than 3 days/prolonged immobility
	   • Increasing age
	   • Laparoscopic surgery
	   • Obesity (BMI > 40)
	   • Varicose veins

Important differential diagnoses	• MSK, tear • Ruptured Baker cyst • Cellulitis • Superficial phlebitis

Deep Vein Thrombosis – cont'd

Potential investigations	• Comparing calf measurement
	• Well's Score
	• FBC
	• U&E
	• CRP
	• Glucose
	• D-Dimer: if Well's score indicates that a DVT is 'unlikely' (1 point or less) then normal D-Dimer rules out DVT
	• Higher level:
	  • Venous doppler ultrasound
	  • Contrast venography
	  • MR venography

Interventions and disposal options[40]	• Refer immediately for same-day assessment and management if suspected in a woman who is pregnant or has given birth within the past 6 weeks
	• DVT likely if Wells score two points or more, and unlikely if score is one point or less
	• DVT likely:
	  • Proximal leg vein ultrasound scan with the results available within 4 h if possible
	  • Otherwise:
	    ◦ Conduct D-dimer test, then
	    ◦ Interim therapeutic anticoagulation, and
	    ◦ USS within 24 h
	• DVT unlikely:
	  • D-dimer test:
	    ◦ If results cannot be obtained within 4 h:
	    ◦ Offer interim therapeutic anticoagulation while awaiting the result
	    ◦ If D-dimer test positive, offer a proximal leg vein ultrasound scan with the results available within 4 h if possible
	  • If results cannot be obtained within 4 h:
	    ◦ Offer interim therapeutic anticoagulation and a proximal leg vein ultrasound scan with the result available within 24 h
	  • If D-dimer test is negative:
	    ◦ Stop interim therapeutic anticoagulation
	    ◦ Consider alternative diagnosis
	    ◦ Explain DVT unlikely and discuss signs and symptoms of DVT, and when and where to seek further medical help
	• Interim therapeutic anticoagulation:
	    ◦ First line: apixaban or rivaroxaban
	    ◦ Second line: LMWH for at least 5 days followed by dabigatran or edoxaban, or LMWH concurrently with a vitamin K antagonist for at least 5 days
	• Conduct baseline blood tests including:
	    ◦ FBC
	    ◦ U&Es
	    ◦ LFTs
	    ◦ Prothrombin time (PT)
	    ◦ Activated partial thromboplastin time (APTT)

Deep Vein Thrombosis

| Special considerations | • Consider PE if the patient has a DVT (manifestations of the same disease process)
• Revised Well's Score (Fig. 7.46):
  • Active cancer (treatment within last 6 months or palliative) (1)
  • Calf swelling ≥3 cm compared to asymptomatic calf (measured 10 cm below tibial tuberosity) (1)
  • Collateral superficial veins (non-varicose) (1)
  • Pitting oedema (confined to symptomatic leg) (1)
  • Swelling of entire leg (1)
  • Localised tenderness along distribution of deep venous system (1)
  • Paralysis, paresis, or recent cast immobilisation of lower extremity (1)
  • Recently bedridden ≥3 days, or major surgery requiring regional or general anaesthetic in the previous 12 weeks (1)
  • Previously documented deep-vein thrombosis (1)
  • Alternative diagnosis at least as likely as DVT (−2)
• Analysis:
  • DVT 'likely' if 2 points or more
  • DVT is 'unlikely' if 1 point or less |

Well's score showing risk factors for deep venous thrombosis (DVT)	
Criteria	**Score**
• Lower limb trauma, surgery, or immobilization in a plaster cast	+1
• Bedridden for more than three days or surgery within last four weeks	+1
• Tenderness along line of femoral or popliteal veins	+1
• Entire limb swollen	+1
• Calf more than 3cm greater in circumference, measured 10 cm below tibial tuberosity	+1
• Pitting oedema	+1
• Dilated collateral superficial veins	+1
• Past history of DVT (confirmed)	+1
• Malignancy	+1
• Intravenous drug use	+3
• Alternative diagnosis more likely than DVT	−2
DVT 'likely if well's >1 DVT 'unlikely if well's <2	

Fig. 7.46 Well's score showing risk factors for deep venous thrombosis (DVT). (From Evans, Newby & Horton-Szar, 2012.)

Pulmonary Embolism

| Classic history | • SOB
• Pleuritic chest pain
• Haemoptysis
• Syncope with cyanosis in massive PE |

Pulmonary Embolism

Classic findings	• Tachycardia • Tachypnoea • Pleural rub • Raised JVP • Cyanosis • Pyrexia • Hypotension (massive PE) • DVT findings

Potential investigations	• D-Dimer:
	  • Patients scoring 2 or more on Well's score OR with elevated D-Dimer require pulmonary imaging
	  • Normal D-Dimer does not exclude PE if moderate or high probability of PE, but negative D-dimer rules out PE with a high predictive value in patients with a low or moderate clinical probability
	• FBC
	• U&Es
	• ECG (sinus tachycardia, classic SI, QIII, TIII with RBBB, consider MI, pericarditis)
	• CXR
	• Higher level:
	  • Ventilation-perfusion scan
	  • CTPA (CT pulmonary angiogram)

Interventions and disposal options	• If PE is presumed:
	  • Vascular access
	  • Admit P1

Special considerations	• Modified Well's Score for PE[41]:
	• Signs of DVT (3.0)
	• IV drug use (3.0)
	• PE is most likely diagnosis (3.0)
	• HR >100 (1.5)
	• Prior PE or DVT (1.5)
	• Bed ridden for >3 days or surgery within 4 weeks (1.5)
	• Cancer treated actively or palliation last 6/12 (1.0)
	• Haemoptysis (1.0)
	• Risk: <2 = low/2–6 = moderate/>6 = high
	• Non-thrombotic causes include emboli from:
	  • Amniotic fluid
	  • Air
	  • Fat
	  • Tumour
	  • Sepsis

Ruptured Abdominal Aortic Aneurysm

Classic history	• Ranges from symptomless to PEA cardiac arrest • Central abdominal pain radiating to back • Features of shock
Classic findings	• Tender pulsatile abdominal mass • Shock – distress, pallor, sweating, tachycardia, hypotension, mottled skin
Important differential diagnoses	• Ureteric colic • General abdominal pain causes (see acute abdomen table)

Ruptured Abdominal Aortic Aneurysm	

UUC interventions and disposal	• Low threshold for considering
	• P1 transfer – pre-alert
	• Ultrasound scan would offer 'rule in', not 'rule out'
	• Once considered:
	  • High flow oxygen
	  • Large bore canula
	  • IV fluids
	  • IV analgesia
	  • IV antiemetic
	  • Catheter

References

1. NICE.. *Sepsis: Recognition, Diagnosis and Early Management*; 2017. https://www.nice.org.uk/guidance/ng51. All rights reserved. Subject to Notice of rights. NICE guidance is prepared for the National Health Service in England. All NICE guidance is subject to regular review and may be updated or withdrawn. NICE accepts no responsibility for the use of its content in this product/publication.

2. NICE. *Suspected Cancer: Recognition and Referral*; 2021. https://www.nice.org.uk/guidance/ng12/chapter/1-Recommendations-organised-by-site-of-cancer. All rights reserved. Subject to Notice of rights. NICE guidance is prepared for the National Health Service in England. All NICE guidance is subject to regular review and may be updated or withdrawn. NICE accepts no responsibility for the use of its content in this product/publication.

3. NICE. *Suspected Cancer: Recognition and Referral*; 2021. https://www.nice.org.uk/guidance/ng12/chapter/1-Recommendations-organised-by-site-of-cancer. All rights reserved. Subject to Notice of rights. NICE guidance is prepared for the National Health Service in England. All NICE guidance is subject to regular review and may be updated or withdrawn. NICE accepts no responsibility for the use of its content in this product/publication.

4. NICE. *Suspected Cancer: Recognition and Referral*; 2021. https://www.nice.org.uk/guidance/ng12/chapter/1-Recommendations-organised-by-site-of-cancer. All rights reserved. Subject to Notice of rights. NICE guidance is prepared for the National Health Service in England. All NICE guidance is subject to regular review and may be updated or withdrawn. NICE accepts no responsibility for the use of its content in this product/publication.

5. NICE. *Suspected Cancer: Recognition and Referral*; 2021. https://www.nice.org.uk/guidance/ng12/chapter/1-Recommendations-organised-by-site-of-cancer. All rights reserved. Subject to Notice of rights. NICE guidance is prepared for the National Health Service in England. All NICE guidance is subject to regular review and may be updated or withdrawn. NICE accepts no responsibility for the use of its content in this product/publication.

6. Antman EM, Cohen M, Bernink P, et al. The TIMI risk score for unstable angina/non–ST elevation MI: a method for prognostication and therapeutic decision making. *JAMA*. 2000;284(7):835–842. https://doi.org/10.1001/jama.284.7.835.

7. DVLA. Assessing fitness to drive – a guide for medical professionals. Accessed 6 January 2021.

8. NICE. *Chronic Heart Failure in Adults: Diagnosis and Management*; 2018. https://www.nice.org.uk/guidance/ng106/chapter/recommendations#didiagnosi-heart-failure. All rights reserved. Subject to Notice of rights. NICE guidance is prepared for the National Health Service in England. All NICE guidance is subject to regular review and may be updated or withdrawn. NICE accepts no responsibility for the use of its content in this product/publication.

9. NICE. *Hypertension in Adults: Diagnosis and Management*; 2019. https://www.nice.org.uk/guidance/ng136/chapter/Recommendations#iidentifyin-who-to-refer-for-same-day-specialist-review. All rights reserved. Subject to Notice of rights. NICE guidance is prepared for the National Health Service in England. All NICE guidance is subject to regular review and may be updated or withdrawn. NICE accepts no responsibility for the use of its content in this product/publication.

10. NICE. *Suspected Cancer: Recognition and Referral*; 2021. https://www.nice.org.uk/guidance/ng12/chapter/1-Recommendations-organised-by-site-of-cancer. All rights reserved. Subject to Notice of rights. NICE guidance is prepared for the National Health Service in England. All NICE guidance is subject to regular review and may be updated or withdrawn. NICE accepts no responsibility for the use of its content in this product/publication.

11. Everett JS, Budescu M, Sommers MS. Making sense of skin color in clinical care. *Clin Nurs Res.* 2012;21(4):495–516. https://doi.org/10.1177/1054773812446510.

12. Lawton S. Assessing the patient with a skin condition. *J Tissue Viability.* 2001;11(3):113–115. https://doi.org/10.1016/S0965-206X(01)80040-1.

13. NICE. *Suspected Cancer: Recognition and Referral*; 2021. https://www.nice.org.uk/guidance/ng12/chapter/1-Recommendations-organised-by-site-of-cancer. All rights reserved. Subject to Notice of rights. NICE guidance is prepared for the National Health Service in England. All NICE guidance is subject to regular review and may be updated or withdrawn. NICE accepts no responsibility for the use of its content in this product/publication.

14. NICE. *Respiratory Tract Infections (Self-Limiting): Prescribing Antibiotics*; 2008. https://www.nice.org.uk/guidance/cg69/chapter/Introduction. All rights reserved. Subject to Notice of rights. NICE guidance is prepared for the National Health Service in England. All NICE guidance is subject to regular review and may be updated or withdrawn. NICE accepts no responsibility for the use of its content in this product/publication.

15. NICE. *Otitis Media (Acute): Antimicrobial Prescribing.* 2018. https://www.nice.org.uk/guidance/ng91. All rights reserved. Subject to Notice of rights. NICE guidance is prepared for the National Health Service in England. All NICE guidance is subject to regular review and may be updated or withdrawn. NICE accepts no responsibility for the use of its content in this product/publication.

16. Centor R, Witherspoon J, Dalton H, et al. The diagnosis of strep throat in adults in the emergency room. *Med Decis Mak.* 1981;1(3):239–246.

17. NICE. *Sore Throat (Acute): Antimicrobial Prescribing*; 2021. https://www.nice.org.uk/guidance/ng84/chapter/terms-used-in-the-guideline. All rights reserved. Subject to Notice of rights. NICE guidance is prepared for the National Health Service in England. All NICE guidance is subject to regular review and may be updated or withdrawn. NICE accepts no responsibility for the use of its content in this product/publication.

18. Greater Manchester Health & Social Care Partnership, Greater Manchester and Eastern Cheshire Strategic Clinical Networks and Greater Manchester Medicines Management Group. *Palliative Care Pain & Symptom Control Guidelines for Adults*; 2019. https://www.england.nhs.uk/north-west/wp-content/uploads/sites/48/2020/01/Palliative-Care-Pain-and-Symptom-Control-Guidelines.pdf. Accessed 27 January 2021. Reproduced with kind permission from the Greater Manchester Medicines Management Group Greater Manchester and Eastern Cheshire Strategic Clinical Networks.

19. Health Improvement Scotland, NHS Scotland. Scottish Palliative Care Guidelines. https://www.palliativecareguidelines.scot.nhs.uk. Accessed 30 January 2021.

20. World Health Organisation. WHO Guidelines for the pharmacological and radiotherapeutic management of cancer pain in adults and adolescents. https://www.who.int/ncds/management/palliative-care/cancer-pain-guidelines/en/. Accessed 30 January 2021.

21. NICE. *Suspected Cancer: Recognition and Referral*; 2021. https://www.nice.org.uk/guidance/ng12/chapter/1-Recommendations-organised-by-site-of-cancer. All rights reserved. Subject to Notice of rights. NICE guidance is prepared for the National Health Service in England. All NICE guidance is subject to regular review and may be updated or withdrawn. NICE accepts no responsibility for the use of its content in this product/publication.

22. NICE. *Suspected Cancer: Recognition and Referral*; 2021. https://www.nice.org.uk/guidance/ng12/chapter/1-Recommendations-organised-by-site-of-cancer. All rights reserved. Subject to Notice of rights. NICE guidance is prepared for the National Health Service in England. All NICE guidance is subject to regular review and may be updated or withdrawn. NICE accepts no responsibility for the use of its content in this product/publication.

23. NICE. *Suspected Cancer: Recognition and Referral*; 2021. https://www.nice.org.uk/guidance/ng12/chapter/1-Recommendations-organised-by-site-of-cancer. All rights reserved. Subject to Notice of rights. NICE guidance is prepared for the National Health Service in England. All NICE guidance is subject to regular review and may be updated or withdrawn. NICE accepts no responsibility for the use of its content in this product/publication.

24. Martínez-Cara JG, Jiménez-Rosales R, Úbeda-Muñoz M, et al. Comparison of AIMS65, Glasgow–Blatchford score, and Rockall score in a European series of patients with upper gastrointestinal

bleeding: performance when predicting in-hospital and delayed mortality. *United European Gastroenterol J.* 2016;4(3):371–379. https://doi.org/10.1177/2050640615604779.

25. NICE. *Suspected Cancer: Recognition and Referral*; 2021. https://www.nice.org.uk/guidance/ng12/chapter/1-Recommendations-organised-by-site-of-cancer. All rights reserved. Subject to Notice of rights. NICE guidance is prepared for the National Health Service in England. All NICE guidance is subject to regular review and may be updated or withdrawn. NICE accepts no responsibility for the use of its content in this product/publication.

26. NICE. *Scenario: Back pain low – (without radiculopathy): Red flag symptoms and signs* 2022. https://cks.nice.org.uk/topics/back-pain-low-without-radiculopathy/diagnosis/red-flag-symptoms-signs/. All rights reserved. Subject to Notice of rights. NICE guidance is prepared for the National Health Service in England. All NICE guidance is subject to regular review and may be updated or withdrawn. NICE accepts no responsibility for the use of its content in this product/publication.

27. Hall A, Aubrey-Bassler K, Thorne B, et al. Do not routinely offer imaging for uncomplicated low back pain. *BMJ.* 2021;372:n291.

28. NICE. *Suspected Cancer: Recognition and Referral*; 2021. https://www.nice.org.uk/guidance/ng12/chapter/1-Recommendations-organised-by-site-of-cancer. All rights reserved. Subject to Notice of rights. NICE guidance is prepared for the National Health Service in England. All NICE guidance is subject to regular review and may be updated or withdrawn. NICE accepts no responsibility for the use of its content in this product/publication.

29. NICE. *Scenario: Managing Someone With Suspected Epilepsy*, 2021. https://cks.nice.org.uk/topics/epilepsy/management/suspected-epilepsy/. All rights reserved. Subject to Notice of rights. NICE guidance is prepared for the National Health Service in England. All NICE guidance is subject to regular review and may be updated or withdrawn. NICE accepts no responsibility for the use of its content in this product/publication.

30. NICE. *Headaches in Over 12s: Diagnosis and Management*; 2015. https://www.nice.org.uk/guidance/cg150. All rights reserved. Subject to Notice of rights. NICE guidance is prepared for the National Health Service in England. All NICE guidance is subject to regular review and may be updated or withdrawn. NICE accepts no responsibility for the use of its content in this product/publication.

31. Goadsby PJ. Recent advances in the diagnosis and management of migraine. *BMJ.* 2006;332(7532):25–29. https://doi.org/10.1136/bmj.332.7532.25.

32. Nor AM, Davis J, Sen B, et al. The Recognition of Stroke in the Emergency Room (ROSIER) scale: development and validation of a stroke recognition instrument. *Lancet Neurol.* 2005;4(11):727–734. https://doi.org/10.1016/S1474-4422(05)70201-5.

33. NICE. *Stroke and Transient Ischaemic Attack in Over 16s: Diagnosis and Initial Management.* 2019. https://www.nice.org.uk/guidance/ng128. All rights reserved. Subject to Notice of rights. NICE guidance is prepared for the National Health Service in England. All NICE guidance is subject to regular review and may be updated or withdrawn. NICE accepts no responsibility for the use of its content in this product/publication.

34. NICE. *Suspected Cancer: Recognition and Referral*; 2021. https://www.nice.org.uk/guidance/ng12/chapter/1-Recommendations-organised-by-site-of-cancer. All rights reserved. Subject to Notice of rights. NICE guidance is prepared for the National Health Service in England. All NICE guidance is subject to regular review and may be updated or withdrawn. NICE accepts no responsibility for the use of its content in this product/publication.

35. NICE. *Menorrhagia*; 2018. https://cks.nice.org.uk/topics/menorrhagia/. All rights reserved. Subject to Notice of rights. NICE guidance is prepared for the National Health Service in England. All NICE guidance is subject to regular review and may be updated or withdrawn. NICE accepts no responsibility for the use of its content in this product/publication.

36. NICE. *Suspected Cancer: Recognition and Referral*; 2021. https://www.nice.org.uk/guidance/ng12/chapter/1-Recommendations-organised-by-site-of-cancer. All rights reserved. Subject to Notice of rights. NICE guidance is prepared for the National Health Service in England. All NICE guidance is subject to regular review and may be updated or withdrawn. NICE accepts no responsibility for the use of its content in this product/publication.

37. McNally M, Curtain J, O'Brien K, et al. Validity of British Thoracic Society guidance (the CRB-65 rule) for predicting the severity of pneumonia in general practice: systematic review and meta-analysis. *Br J Gen Pract.* 2010;60(579):e423–e433. https://doi.org/10.3399/bjgp10X532422.

38. NICE. *Pneumonia (Community-Acquired): Antimicrobial Prescribing*; 2020. https://www.nice.org.uk/guidance/ng138/chapter/Recommendations#treatment-for-adults-young-people-and-children. All rights reserved. Subject to Notice of rights. NICE guidance is prepared for the National Health Service

in England. All NICE guidance is subject to regular review and may be updated or withdrawn. NICE accepts no responsibility for the use of its content in this product/publication.

39. NICE. *Suspected Cancer: Recognition and Referral*; 2021. https://www.nice.org.uk/guidance/ng12/chapter/1-Recommendations-organised-by-site-of-cancer. All rights reserved. Subject to Notice of rights. NICE guidance is prepared for the National Health Service in England. All NICE guidance is subject to regular review and may be updated or withdrawn. NICE accepts no responsibility for the use of its content in this product/publication.

40. NICE. *Deep Vein Thrombosis*; 2020. https://cks.nice.org.uk/topics/deep-vein-thrombosis/. All rights reserved. Subject to Notice of rights. NICE guidance is prepared for the National Health Service in England. All NICE guidance is subject to regular review and may be updated or withdrawn. NICE accepts no responsibility for the use of its content in this product/publication.

41. NICE. *Pulmonary Embolism*; 2020. Available from https://cks.nice.org.uk/topics/pulmonary-embolism/. All rights reserved. Subject to Notice of rights. NICE guidance is prepared for the National Health Service in England. All NICE guidance is subject to regular review and may be updated or withdrawn. NICE accepts no responsibility for the use of its content in this product/publication.

42. Semple D, Smyth R. 2019. Oxford Handbook of Psychiatry. Oxford: Oxford University Press, Incorporated.

43. Ralston S, Penman I, Strachan M, Hobson R. *Davidson's Principles and Practice of Medicine*. 23rd ed. 2018.

44. Urden L, Stacy K, Lough M. *Priorities in Critical Care Nursing*. 8th ed. 2020.

45. Feather A, Randall D, Waterhouse M. *Kumar and Clark's Clinical Medicine*. 10th ed. 2021.

46. Zenith. *Medical Assistant: Digestive System, Nutrition, Financial Management and First AidR—Module C*. 2nd ed. 2016.

47. Flynn TR. Surgical management of orofacial infections. *Atlas Oral Maxillofac Surg. Clin. North Am*. 8:79, 2000.

48. Rao S, Rao K. *Essentials of Surgery for Dental Students*. 1st ed. 2016.

49. Scully C. Medical problems in dentistry. 6th ed. *Norwalk*. 2010. Churchill Livingstone.

50. Dinulos J. *Habif's Clinical Dermatology*. 7th ed. 2021.

51. Cooper K, Gosnell K. Adult health nursing. 9th ed. 2023.

52. Cohen BA. *Atlas of Pediatric Dermatology*. 4th ed. China:Elsevier Limited. 2013:77.

53. Pizzorno J, Murray M. *Textbook of Natural Medicine*. 5th ed. 2021.

54. Paller AS, Mancini AJ. Hurwitz clinical pediatric dermatology: a textbook of skin disorders of childhood and adolescence. 5th ed. Philadelphia: Elsevier. 2016.

55. James WD, Berger T, Elston DMD. Andrews' diseases of the skin. 11th ed. Philadelphia. 2011. Saunders.

56. High W, Prok LD. *Dermatology Secrets*. 6th ed. 2021.

57. Dockery G, Coughlin M, Crawford M, Hansen ST. *Lower Extremity Soft Tissue & Cutaneous Plastic Surgery*. 2nd ed. 2012.

58. Klatt EC. Robbins y Cotran. Atlas de anatomía patológica, 4th ed. 2022.

59. Brinster N, Liu V, Diwan H, McKee P. *Dermatopathology: High-Yield Pathology*. 1st ed. 2011.

60. Paller A, Mancini A. *Hurwitz Clinical Pediatric Dermatology*. 4th ed. Philadelphia: Elsevier. 2011.

61. Shiland B. *Mastering Healthcare Terminology*. 6th ed. 2019.

62. Jarvis C. Physical examination and health assessment. 7th ed. St. Louis. 2015. Elsevier.

63. Raftery A, Lim E, Ostor A. *Churchill's Pocketbook of Differential Diagnosis*. 4th ed. 2014.

64. Damjanov I, Linder J. Pathology: a color atlas. St. Louis. 1999. Mosby.

65. Mir MA. Atlas of clinical diagnosis, 2nd ed. Edinburgh: Saunders. 2003.

66. Swartz MH. *Textbook of Physical Diagnosis, History and Examination*. 7th ed. 2014.

67. Dhillon R, East CA. Ear, nose and throat and head and neck surgery: an illustrated colour text. 4th ed. 2012.

68. Neville B, Damm DD, Allen C, Bouquot J. Oral and maxillofacial pathology. 3rd ed. 2009.

69. De M, Anari S. Infections and foreign bodies in ENT. MPSUR (ISSN: 0263-9319). October 2018.

70. Waldman S. *Pain Review*. 2nd ed. 2017.

71. Kumar P, Clark M. *Kumar & Clark's Medical Management and Therapeutics*. 1st ed. 2011.

72. Adappa R, Hewitt M. Applied knowledge in paediatrics: MRCPCH mastercourse. 1st ed. 2022.

73. Patton KT. Anatomy and physiology. 10th ed. St. Louis. Elsevier. 2019.

74. Evans J, Newby DE, Horton-Szar D. *Crash Course: Cardiovascular System*. 4th ed. 2012.

The Diploma in Urgent Medical Care

The Diploma in Urgent Medical Care

Examination Outline

Those intending to undertake the Royal College of Surgeons of Edinburgh's Diploma in Urgent Medical Care (DUMC) should fully familiarise themselves with the examination's guidelines and regulations available on the College website.[1]

The DUMC examination is comprised of a 180 single best answer (SBA) paper and 12 structured oral questions set at a level to ensure patient safety and allow the candidate to demonstrate a level of knowledge expected of a level 7 practitioner or above (as described in the Skills for Health framework).[2] Greater success is likely to be derived by applying a pragmatic approach based on experience in the 'real world'. Questions are based on UK practice and guidelines and can be drawn from any area deemed to be covered by the examination syllabus according to the distribution shown in Table 8.1:

TABLE 8.1 ■ Indicative Distribution of Questions

Syllabus Area	Percentage (%)
Working in Urgent Medical Systems	10
Practising Urgent Medical Care	40
Using Technology in Urgent Care	7.5
Managing Safe Dispositions	10
Risk Management	7.5
Urgent Care Preparedness	7.5
Operational Practice (cross-cutting theme)	7.5
Human Factors (cross-cutting theme)	10

Example Single Best Answer (SBA) Questions

The SBA format is widely used in undergraduate and postgraduate medical examinations. You will typically be presented with:
- A clinical scenario or vignette which sets the scene
- A 'lead-in' question which refers to the scenario
- A list of possible responses from which you must choose the single *best* or most likely answer

By their nature, these questions can be long and time-consuming. This may be considered a good thing, as examiners will aim to include relevant material in the scenario that should help identify the correct answer. However, be prepared to read through material quickly in order to avoid time constraints. Importantly, unlike other multiple-choice question (MCQ) formats, it may be that a number of answers *could* be true; the key is to choose the single best answer or that which is *most likely* to be correct. This often means selecting pragmatic, 'real world' clinical decisions rather than erring on a risk-averse approach.

EXAMPLE QUESTION 1

You are the clinical lead for a company tendering to run a new urgent treatment centre (UTC). Your manager asks you to assist in putting together a bid. Which of the following would be the best advice to give?
   a. The UTC must be open 24 hours a day
   b. The UTC must be GP-led but can be staffed by GPs, nurses and other clinicians
   c. The UTC must offer FAST scanning to rule out intra-abdominal pathology
   d. The UTC would divert all minor ailments back to the GP
   e. The UTC would work in isolation from other parts of the locally integrated urgent and emergency care system

Answer a: is incorrect because UTCs must be open at least 12 hours a day
Answer b: is CORRECT because according to NHSE, UTC's must be GP-led but can be staffed by GPs, nurses and other clinicians
Answer c: is incorrect. UTCs must offer a number a variety of investigations, but they do not include FAST scanning
Answer d: is incorrect as UTCs would manage minor ailments
Answer e: is incorrect as UTCs would work as part of the locally integrated urgent and emergency care system

EXAMPLE QUESTION 2

You are a clinician working in an UTC where you see a 24-year-old woman who has suffered very heavy, painful periods for the past 10 months. Her latest period started yesterday; she is pale and tired and requests help, as she has been unable to visit her GP. Which of the following course of action would be most appropriate?
   a. Advise her to see her GP as this is a primary care problem
   b. Suggest she start an oral contraceptive so long as she is not trying to conceive
   c. Check her full blood count and recommend she starts tranexamic acid now and books to see her GP
   d. Arrange for her to undergo investigations including FBC, clotting, U&E, LFT, ferritin, hormone profile and TFTs
   e. Arrange a smear, swabs and ultrasound to help determine the source of excess bleeding

Answer a: is incorrect because, while menorrhagia should be assessed, investigated and treated by primary care, you still have a role in managing this particular UUC presentation
Answer b: is incorrect because, while oral contraceptives may be used to manage menorrhagia, they are not typically a first line treatment and the patient's GP would commence such treatment
Answer c: is CORRECT because it would be appropriate to check the FBC in this circumstance to exclude serious anaemia and tranexamic acid would be a good first line treatment to manage symptoms while the patient arranges to discuss further with her GP
Answer d: is incorrect because, while all these blood tests might form part of an assessment for menorrhagia, they would be performed by her GP
Answer e: is incorrect because, while all these blood tests might be reasonable depending on history and physical findings, they should typically be performed by her GP

EXAMPLE QUESTION 3

As the clinical lead in an UTC, you are trying to manage the frustrations of some staff who feel patients are attending inappropriately. Which of the following statements would be correct?

a. The problem is all to do with 'inappropriate attendance'.

b. Most people use urgent care services all the time.

c. There may be a link between volume of A&E attendance and hospital admissions

d. It would be helpful if commissioners increased the frequency at which out of hours were re-commissioned.

e. It is best just to block frequent attendees at the front door.

Answer a: is incorrect because, while a small group of users may consistently use the system in a different way from most, the majority of patients use the services appropriately, given the patients' perceived urgency at the time of use

Answer b: is incorrect because most people use the urgent care system rarely (on average once every six years for out-of-hours and A&E every three years)

Answer c: is CORRECT because there is some evidence that when A&E departments become overwhelmed junior staff will admit more people – the primary failure is in the A&E system, not the volume presenting

Answer d: is incorrect, because tender cycles which are too frequent may reduce levels of care since they make it difficult for a provider to invest, are expensive and may lead to focus on price rather than quality and patient safety

Answer e: is incorrect because every patient presenting to an urgent and unscheduled care service should be clinically assessed regardless of previous presenting patterns

Example Structured Oral Questions

Structured oral questions are recognised by the Joint Committee on Intercollegiate Examinations as one of the best ways to assess knowledge on subject matter through a prepared discussion.

The format involves multiple 'stations' through which the candidate cycles. Typically, each station involves the pre-reading of a scenario and supporting information before sitting down with examiners who progress through a series of prepared questions that aim to test depth of knowledge in pre-determined areas. Such a format reduces the potential bias that is more likely in other oral formats and, importantly, enables assessment of higher-level skills such as knowledge, comprehension, application, analysis, synthesis and evaluation of UUC matters.

Structured oral questions can cover all areas of the syllabus (including clinical, system and managerial). It is recommended that you try to apply an appropriate 'framework' when answering them to ensure that you capture all elements in a comprehensive fashion and demonstrate an ordered rather than 'shotgun' approach.

For example, a clinical area dealing with causes of abdominal discomfort may be dealt with thoroughly either by applying the surgical sieve:

- Autoimmune
- Congenital
- Trauma
- Infection
- Vascular
- Endocrine
- Environment
- Metabolic
- Inflammatory
- Neoplastic

- Degenerative, etc.

Or, otherwise, by considering different clinical areas or groupings, that is:

- Gastroenterological
- Gynaecological
- Genito-urinary
- Musculoskeletal

In the same way, a question dealing with business continuity policy might be approached using a suitable framework:

- Infrastructure (building damage/fire/flooding)
- Equipment (blood machines, radiology)
- Logistics (utilities/fuel)
- Staff (sickness/recruiting/retention/access)
- Information technology (IT; systems loss)
- Demand surge (major incident/system escalation/loss of neighbouring service)

The key to navigating these questions is to construct reasoned, sensible answers which are appropriate, safe, comprehensive and demonstrate maturity in managing to consider the patient of the system as a whole.

EXAMPLE QUESTION 1

Pre-Reading

You are a team leader for an out-of-hours provider. A colleague, Karen, approaches you to raise concerns regarding one of the clinical team members, Mark.

Karen was talking to Mark about a patient he saw on last night's shift, and she thinks he may have prescribed the wrong antibiotic. She thinks this is partly due to Mark trying to juggle two separate roles and she is concerned that he is struggling with fatigue.

Question a: Why might you be worried about fatigue amongst your staff?

Fatigue is directly related to:

- Patient safety
- Accidents
- Injuries
- Ill health
- Slower reactions
- Reduced ability to process information
- Memory lapses
- Absent-mindedness
- Decreased awareness
- Lack of attention
- Underestimation of risk, reduced coordination
- Reduced productivity

Question b: What sort of factors might contribute to fatigue?

Individual:

- Age
- Health
- Medication
- Stress
- Sleep loss and/or disruption of the internal clock
- External factors (working too much)

Work:

- Excessive work, prolonged hours, juggling commitments

- Poorly designed shift-working arrangements including night shifts
- Inadequate with time for rest and recovery
- Prolonged physical activity
- Type of work

Question c: How might you address this particular situation?

Mark:

- Concerns have been raised but we do not know whether they are valid
- Explore what he thinks
- Understand his other commitments – are they safe/compatible?
- Discuss this particular consultation and its outcomes
- Examine the medical record
- Audit other patients seen

The patient:

- Confirm whether there has been a clinical error
- Duty of candour - inform and discuss with patient
- Consider clinical situation and outcomes; does a different antibiotic need to be prescribed?

Organisational:

- Significant event
- Potential serious untoward incident (SUI) based on outcomes?
- Consider HR policies – has there been a breach?
- Whistleblowing policy – affects Karen
- Duty of candour
- Potential disciplinary process
- Potential training / education outcomes
- Audit clinical activity

EXAMPLE QUESTION 2

Pre-Reading

You are a clinician working in an UTC where the clinical lead asks you to contribute to the re-write of the unit's business continuity plan.

Question a: Which external organisations have an interest in knowing your centre has a robust business continuity plan?

Other local healthcare providers, including:

- General practices
- Acute trusts
- Out-of-hours providers
- The CCG
- The CQC

Question b: What sort of issues could interrupt business and clinical activity?

Infrastructure:

- Building damage
- Fire, flooding
- Loss of critical equipment – that is scanners, blood machines

Logistics:

- Loss of utilities/fuel
- Resupply
- Ordering systems
- Weather

Staff:
- Sickness
- Recruiting and retention crises
- Access (weather)

IT:
- Loss of capability
  Patients:
- Surges in demand
- Major incident
- System escalation
- Loss of neighbouring service

Question c: What sort of things might a business continuity plans contain?
- Articulation of essential 'capability'
- Important communications/contacts list
- Risk assessments
- Actions on major incidents/system escalation
- Staff roles in an incident
- How to keep essential services functioning
- Initial action cards
- Key premises details
- Plans for move to alternative premises

EXAMPLE QUESTION 3

Pre-Reading

You are conducting an out-of-hours shift on the Friday of a Bank Holiday weekend when you are called to conduct a home visit on a 68-year-old man who has been coughing up bright red blood for 8 hours. When you arrive, he looks thin, unwell and pale but all his observations are normal.
Question a: What sort of conditions might cause haemoptysis?
Respiratory:
- Neoplasm
- Infection (lower respiratory tract infection [LRTI], tuberculosis)
- Bronchiectasis

Cardiovascular:
- Pulmonary embolism
- Pulmonary oedema
- Coagulation disorder
- Trauma

Ear, nose and throat:
- Nosebleeds and related

Other:
- Mitral stenosis
- Wegener's granulomatosis

Question b: What history and clinical findings would support a diagnosis of pulmonary embolism?
History:
- Shortness of breath
- Pleuritic chest pain
- Haemoptysis
- Syncope with cyanosis (in massive pulmonary embolism [PE])

Clinical findings:
- Tachycardia
- Tachypnoea
- Pleural rub
- Raised jugular venous pressure (JVP)
- Cyanosis
- Pyrexia
- Hypotension (massive PE)
- Deep vein thrombosis (DVT) findings
- ECG (sinus tachycardia, classic SI, QIII, TIII with right bundle branch block [RBBB])

Question c: You are concerned, despite this patient's normal observations, that his history and appearance warrant urgent review either at a local UTC or at a district general hospital. Which investigations (relevant to haemoptysis of unknown origin) might be available at each of these sites?

Urgent treatment centre:
- Full blood count, coagulation, U&Es, LFTs
- Arterial blood gas
- D-dimer
- Chest x-ray (CXR)
- ECG
- Urinalysis
- Sputum M, C and S

District General Hospital – all the above plus:
- CP pulmonary angiogram (CTPA) / Ventilation/perfusion scan (PE)
- CT Scan
- Bronchoscopy

EXAMPLE QUESTION 4

Pre-Reading

You are asked to conduct a home visit to a 49-year-old lady who is known to have late-stage metastatic breast cancer and struggles to look after herself. Over the last week she has developed malaise, weakness and thirst which seem out of keeping from her preceding experience.

Question a: Which teams might have regular contact with a patient with this condition?

Primary care:
- GP
- Nurse
- Visiting team

Secondary care:
- Breast surgeon
- Oncology
- Palliative care nurse

Community care:
- District nurses
- Intermediate care teams

Cancer care:
- Hospice
- Palliative care nurses

- MacMillan
- Marie Curie

Charity, examples being:

- Breast Cancer UK
- Pink Ribbon Foundation
- Breast Cancer Haven

Social care:

- Adult social care

Question b: What could account for this patient's symptoms of malaise, weakness and thirst?

Cancer-related complications:

- Hypercalcaemia
- Disease progression
- Anxiety and depression

Non-cancer related:

- Intercurrent illness
- Dehydration
- Neglect (poor intake, difficulty with self-care including shopping and cooking)

Question c: What related clinical features would suggest this may be due to hypercalcaemia?

Common symptoms:

- Malaise
- Weakness
- Anorexia
- Thirst
- Nausea
- Constipation

More severe symptoms:

- Vomiting
- Ileus
- Delirium
- Seizures
- Drowsiness
- Coma

Question d: You consider this patient's symptoms may be due to hypercalcaemia. What are your management options?

Discuss with patient (explaining this complication can be relatively easily corrected)

Active management:

- Biochemical assessment (corrected calcium, U&Es, eGFR, LFTs)
- Seek immediate specialist advice

Further treatment options depend on advice and calcium levels but may include:

- Whether first or recurring
- Prognosis and prior quality of life
- Patient's consent to iv treatment and tests
- Medication changes
- IV fluids
- IV bisphosphonate

Palliative care management:

- Involve wider palliative care team
- Symptom management

EXAMPLE QUESTION 5

Pre-Reading

You are preparing a tutorial aimed at teaching new clinicians about laboratory investigations that may be particularly useful in the urgent and unscheduled care environment.

Question a: What range of testing might be available via UTCs?

Haematology:

- FBC

Biochemistry:

- U&Es
- LFTs
- Amylase
- D-Dimer
- Arterial blood gas / venous blood gas
- Troponin

Microbiology

- M, C and S (urine, swabs, sputum)

Near-patient:

- Urine dipstick
- Pregnancy test
- Blood glucose

Radiology:

- Bladder scan
- X-ray
- Ultrasound (including FAST scanning)

Question b: How would you explain C-Reactive Protein (CRP)?

- Acute phase reactant
- A protein made by the liver and released into the blood within a few hours after tissue injury (examples causes include infection, inflammation, myocardial infarction, sepsis, late-stage pregnancy, women taking hormone replacement therapy [HRT], obesity)
- *Not* diagnostic: must be used in conjunction with other factors (signs, symptoms, examination, additional investigations)
- Blood levels less than 10 mg/L are unlikely to be clinically significant
- Classically a delayed 'response' – levels rise rapidly within the first 6 to 8 hours and peak after 48 hours
- CRP concentration rises and falls faster than ESR

Question c: How would you describe D-Dimer?

- One of the fibrin degradation products from disintegrating clots, normally undetectable
- Significant negative predictive value in excluding venous blood clots especially in low-risk patients
- No 'positive predictive value' – it is raised in many conditions and does not help to narrow down a differential diagnosis if positive
- Helps exclude, diagnose, and monitor diseases and conditions that cause hypercoagulability, that is DVT, pulmonary embolism, disseminated intravascular coagulation
- False positives may be associated with recent surgery, trauma, infection, liver or kidney disease, cancers, normal pregnancy and some diseases of pregnancy, that is eclampsia, the elderly, rheumatoid arthritis, red blood cell rupture (including improper collection and handling)

- False negative value may follow anticoagulation therapy
- Hospital laboratory results are mostly quantitative; near-patient are mostly qualitative

Question d: How would you describe D-Dimer?

- One of the proteins in muscle fibres that help regulate muscle contraction
- Three different troponins: skeletal muscle troponin C (TnC) and two heart muscle troponins, cardiac troponin T (cTnT) and cardiac troponin I (cTnI)
- Historically: standard cTnI or cTnT test
- Now: high-sensitivity troponins (hs-cTnI or hs-cTnT) detect highly specific marker of heart damage at very low levels
- Biochemical diagnosis of acute heart muscle damage requires an increase in the troponin concentration with time
- If a patient with chest pain and known stable angina has a normal and stable hs-cTn troponin result, it is likely that their heart has not been damaged
- Diagnosis requires combination of biochemical result, physical examination, clinical history and ECG
- False variable positives (of MI) include myocarditis, acute heart failure, arrhythmia, chest injury, stroke, PE or pulmonary embolism
- False constant positives (of MI) include chronic heart failure, hypertension, kidney disease, severe infections and chronic inflammatory muscle conditions

EXAMPLE QUESTION 6

Pre-Reading

You are conducting an out of hours shift when you are called to perform a home visit on a 52-year-old woman who has been generally unwell for 2 days and now appears to be hyperventilating. She has been passing more urine than normal, feels parched and has a 'racing heart'. Her family say she has funny breath, and they are very worried about her.

Question a: What are the common medical (non-trauma) causes of hyperventilation?

Respiratory:

- Infection
- Asthma
- COPD
- Pleural effusion
- Haemothorax
- Pneumothorax
- Interstitial lung disease

Cardiac:

- Pulmonary oedema
- Acute coronary syndrome (ACS)
- PE
- Arrythmia including fast atrial fibrillation (AF)

Systemic/other:

- Pyrexia
- Anaemia
- Hypovolaemia
- Anxiety/stress/'hyperventilation'
- Diabetic keto-acidosis (DKA)
- Hyperthyroidism

Question b: You are concerned that this may be a case of diabetic keto-acidosis. What signs and symptoms might a newly presenting DKA patient present with?

Signs of dehydration:

- Thirst
- Polydipsia
- Polyuria
- Decreased skin turgor
- Dry mouth
- Hypotension
- Tachycardia

GI features:

- Nausea
- Vomiting
- Abdominal pain

Hyperventilation:

- Deep rapid (Kussmaul) breathing
- Acetone breath

Altered consciousness up to coma

Question c: Having identified a DKA crisis in these circumstances, what are the main principles of trying to manage it?

These patients are very unwell and need expert care as soon as possible

Requires Priority 1 (P1) transfer with pre-alert

Initial care may involve:

- ABC
- Oxygen
- IV fluids (0.9% saline)

Higher level care may involve:

- Insulin infusion
- Managing electrolyte imbalance
- Naso-gastric (NG) tube
- Catheter
- Treating infection
- Managing clotting
- Admission to most appropriate area (from acute medical unit [AMU] to intensive care unit [ITU])

EXAMPLE QUESTION 7

Pre-Reading

You are working in an UTC when you are asked to see a 42-year-old lady with a 6-hour history of general right sided abdominal pain.

Question a: What general causes might exist for these symptoms in a woman of her age?

Surgical:

- Appendicitis
- Cholecystitis
- Pancreatitis
- Peptic ulcer, perforation
- Ruptured abdominal aortic aneurysm (AAA)

- Mesenteric infarction
- Diverticulitis
- Large bowel perforation
- Intestinal obstruction
- Renal calculi
- Urinary retention
- Intussusception
- Neoplasm

Gynaecological:

- Ectopic pregnancy
- Pelvic inflammatory disease
- Ovarian cyst including rupture and torsion
- Endometriosis

Medical:

- Acute coronary syndrome
- Pneumonia
- Gastro-oesophageal reflux disease (GORD)
- Diverticulitis
- Pulmonary embolus
- Aortic dissection
- Hepatitis
- Diabetic ketoacidosis
- Urinary tract infection
- Pyelonephritis
- Herpes zoster
- Irritable bowel syndrome
- Inflammatory bowel disease
- Gastroenteritis
- Non-organic

Question b: The patient reports her pain started suddenly 6 hours previously, affecting the right iliac fossa and radiating to her right shoulder. Her last menstrual period was 6 weeks ago, and a pregnancy test is positive. What other risk factors in her history would increase concerns regarding ectopic pregnancy?

- Pelvic inflammatory disease
- Adhesions
- Previous ectopic
- Endometriosis
- Assisted conception
- Intra-uterine contraceptive device (IUCD)
- Progestogen-only pill (POP)
- Congenital abnormalities
- Ovarian/ uterine tumours

Question c: You are concerned this patient may have an ectopic pregnancy; how would you progress the situation?

- Oxygen
- Large bore cannula
- IV fluids
- Analgesia
- P1 transfer with pre-alert

References

1. The Royal College of Surgeons of Edinburgh. Exams. https://www.rcsed.ac.uk/exams. Accessed May 24, 2020.
2. Skills for Health. *Statutory/mandatory core skills training framework (CSTF)*. https://www.skillsforhealth. org.uk/services/item/146-core-skills-training-framework. Accessed May 24, 2020.

Accenture. Accenture 2019 digital health consumer survey. Available at: https://www.accenture.com/_acnmedia/PDF-98/Accenture-2019-Digital-Health-Consumer-Survey-ENG.pdf#zoom=50. Accessed 24 May 2020.

Adamson J, Ben-Shlomo Y, Chaturvedi N, et al. Exploring the impact of patient views on 'appropriate' use of services and help seeking: a mixed method study. *Br J Gen Pract.* 2009;59(564):226. https://doi.org/10.3399/bjgp09X453530.

Antman EM, Cohen M, Bernink PJ, et al. The TIMI risk score for unstable angina/non–ST elevation MI: a method for prognostication and therapeutic decision making. *JAMA.* 2000;284(7):835–842. https://doi.org/10.1001/jama.284.7.835.

Aviation Accidents. *CRM.* Available at: http://www.aviation-accidents.net/tag/crm/page/3/. Accessed 24 May 2020.

Baier N, Geissler A, Bech M, et al. Emergency and urgent care systems in Australia, Denmark, England, France, Germany and the Netherlands – analyzing organization, payment and reforms. *Health Policy.* 2019;123(1):1–10. https://doi.org/10.1016/j.healthpol.2018.11.001.

Balla J, Heneghan C, Thompson M, et al. Clinical decision making in a high-risk primary care environment: a qualitative study in the UK. *BMJ Open.* 2012;2(1):e000414. https://doi.org/10.1136/bmjopen-2011-000414.

Breckman B. The naked consultation – a practical guide to primary care consultation skills. *Nurs Stand.* 2007;21(40):30. https://doi.org/10.7748/ns.21.40.30.s36.

Burchill C. Critical incident stress debriefing: helpful, harmful, or neither? *J Emerg Nurs.* 2019;45(6):611–612. https://doi.org/10.1016/j.jen.2019.08.006.

Care Quality Commission (a). The state of care in independent online primary health services: findings from CQC's programme of comprehensive inspections in England. Available at: https://www.cqc.org.uk/sites/default/files/20180322_state-of-care-independent-online-primary-health-services.pdf. Accessed 24 May 2020.

Care Quality Commission (b). The state of care in urgent primary care services. Available at: https://www.cqc.org.uk/sites/default/files/20180619%20State%20of%20care%20in%20urgent%20primary%20care%20services.pdf. Accessed 24 May 2020.

Care Quality Commission (c). *Briefing: Learning From Serious Incidents in NHS Acute Hospitals: A Review of the Quality of Investigation Reports.* Available at: https://www.cqc.org.uk/sites/default/files/20160608_learning_from_harm_briefing_paper.pdf. Accessed 24 May 2020.

Care Quality Commission (d). *Clarification of Regulatory Methodology: PMS Digital Healthcare Providers.* Available at: https://www.cqc.org.uk/sites/default/files/20170303_pms-digital-healthcare_regulatory-guidance.pdf. Accessed 24 May 2020.

Care Quality Commission (e). The state of care in urgent primary care services. Available at: https://www.cqc.org.uk/sites/default/files/20180619%20State%20of%20care%20in%20urgent%20primary%20care%20services.pdf. Accessed 24 May 2020.

Centor RM, Witherspoon JM, Dalton HP, et al. The diagnosis of strep throat in adults in the emergency room. *Med Decis Making.* 1981;1(3):239–246.

Deloitte. Closing the digital gap | Shaping the future of UK healthcare. Accessed 24 May 2020.

Department for Education, UK Council for Internet Safety, Home Office, et al. Safeguarding children. Available at: https://www.gov.uk/topic/schools-colleges-childrens-services/safeguarding-children. Accessed 24 May 2020.

Department of Health and Social Care. Domestic abuse: a resource for health professionals. Available at: https://www.gov.uk/government/publications/domestic-abuse-a-resource-for-health-professionals. Accessed 24 May 2020.

Department of Health and Social Care. Statutory guidance: care and support statutory guidance. Available at: https://www.gov.uk/government/publications/care-act-statutory-guidance/care-and-support-statutory-guidance. Accessed 24 May 2020.

Donald F, Mohide EA, DiCenso A, et al. Nurse practitioner and physician collaboration in long-term care homes: survey results. *Can J Aging*. 2009;28(1):77–87. https://doi.org/10.1017/S0714980809090060.

Drugs for the doctor's bag: 1-adults. *Drug Ther Bull*. 2015;53(5):56. doi: https://doi.org/10.1136/dtb.2015.5.0328.

Drugs for the doctor's bag: 2-children. *Drug Ther Bull*. 2015;53(6):69. doi: https://doi.org/10.1136/dtb.2015.6.0334.

DVLA. Assessing fitness to drive – a guide for medical professionals. Accessed 6 January 2021. https://assets.publishing.service.gov.uk/government/uploads/system/uploads/attachment_data/file/1084397/assessing-fitness-to-drive-may-2022.pdf

Edrees H, Federico F. *Supporting Clinicians After Medical Error*. London: British Medical Journal Publishing Group; 2015.

Ellis J, Boger E, Latter S, et al. Conceptualisation of the 'good' self-manager: a qualitative investigation of stakeholder views on the self-management of long-term health conditions. *Soc Sci Med*. 2017;176:25–33. https://doi.org/10.1016/j.socscimedw.2017.01.018.

Everett JS, Budescu M, Sommers MS. Making sense of skin color in clinical care. *Clin Nurs Res*. 2012;21(4):495–516. https://doi.org/10.1177/1054773812446510.

Foley C, Droog E, Boyce M, et al. *Patient Experience of Different Regional Models of Urgent and Emergency Care: a Cross-Sectional Survey Study*. London: British Medical Journal Publishing Group; 2017.

General Medical Council. Caring for doctors Caring for patients. Available at: https://www.gmc-uk.org/-/media/documents/caring-for-doctors-caring-for-patients_pdf-80706341.pdf. Accessed 24 May 2020.

Giménez-Espert MDC, Valero-Moreno S, Prado-Gascó VJ. Evaluation of emotional skills in nursing using regression and QCA models: a transversal study. *Nurse Educ Today*. 74:31–37. doi:10.1016/j.nedt.2018.11.019.

Goadsby PJ. Recent advances in the diagnosis and management of migraine. *BMJ*. 2006;332(7532):25–29. https://doi.org/10.1136/bmj.332.7532.25.

Goode J, Hanlon G, Luff D, et al. Male callers to NHS direct: the assertive carer, the new dad and the reluctant patient. *Health (London)*. 2004;8(3):311–328. https://doi.org/10.1177/1363459304043468.

GoodSAM. *GoodSAM*. Available at: https://www.goodsamapp.org. Accessed 24 May 2020.

Gov.uk. Notifiable diseases and causative organisms: how to report. Available at: https://www.gov.uk/guidance/notifiable-diseases-and-causative-organisms-how-to-report. Accessed 28 December 2020.

Greenberg N, Langston V, Jones N. *Trauma Risk Management (TRiM) in the UK Armed Forces*. London: British Medical Journal Publishing Group; 2008.

Hall AM, Aubrey-Bassler K, Thorne B, et al. Do not routinely offer imaging for uncomplicated low back pain. *BMJ*. 2021;372:n291.

Health and Safety Executive (a). Human factors: fatigue. Available at: https://www.hse.gov.uk/humanfactors/topics/fatigue.htm. Accessed 24 May 2020.

Health and Safety Executive (b). Human factors: fatigue. Available at: https://www.hse.gov.uk/humanfactors/topics/fatigue.htm. Accessed 25 October 2020.

Health Improvement Scotland, NHS Scotland. Scottish palliative care guidelines. Available at: https://www.palliativecareguidelines.scot.nhs.uk. Accessed 30 January 2021.

Henderson R. *Monitoring the NHS*. Available at: https://patient.info/doctor/monitoring-the-nhs. Accessed 24 May 2020.

Home Office. Channel guidance. Available at: https://www.gov.uk/government/publications/channel-guidance. Accessed 24 May 2020.

Hootsuite. The global state of digital in 2019. Available at: https://hootsuite.com/en-gb/resources/digital-in-2019. Accessed 24 May 2020.

Houston AM, Pickering AJ. Do I don't I call the doctor': a qualitative study of parental perceptions of calling the GP out-of-hours. *Health Expect.* 2000;3(4):234–242. https://doi.org/10.1046/j.1369-6513.2000.00109.x.

Hughes R. *Patient Safety and Quality: An Evidence-Based Handbook for Nurses.* Rockville, MD: Agency for Healthcare Research and Quality; 2008.

Intercollegiate Board for Training in Pre-hospital Emergency Medicine. Sub-specialty training in pre-hospital emergency medicine: curriculum and assessment system. Available at: http://www.ibtphem.org.uk/media/1039/sub-specialty-training-in-phem-curriculum-assessment-system-edition-2-2015.pdf. Accessed 24 May 2020.

Jackson CJ, Dixon-Woods M, Hsu R, et al. A qualitative study of choosing and using an NHS Walk-in Centre. *Fam Pract.* 2005;22(3):269–274. https://doi.org/10.1093/fampra/cmi018.

Klein JG. *Five Pitfalls in Decisions About Diagnosis and Prescribing.* London: British Medical Journal Publishing Group; 2005.

Lawton S. Assessing the patient with a skin condition. *J Tissue Viability.* 2001;11(3):113–115. https://doi.org/10.1016/S0965-206X(01)80040-1.

Lupton D. *Risk.* 2nd ed. London: Routledge; 2013.

Mackway-Jones K. *Major Incident Medical Management and Support: The Practical Approach at the Scene.* 2nd ed. London: BMJ Books; 2002.

Martínez-Cara JG, Jiménez-Rosales R, Úbeda-Muñoz M, et al. Comparison of AIMS65, Glasgow–Blatchford score, and Rockall score in a European series of patients with upper gastrointestinal bleeding: performance when predicting in-hospital and delayed mortality. *United European Gastroenterol J.* 2016;4(3):371–379. https://doi.org/10.1177/2050640615604779.

McCaig R. Human factors in healthcare: level one. *Occup Med.* 2014;64(7):563. https://doi.org/10.1093/occmed/kqu131.

McGuckin M, Storr J, Longtin Y, et al. Patient empowerment and multimodal hand hygiene promotion: a win-win Strategy. *Am J Med Qual.* 2011;26(1):10–17. https://doi.org/10.1177/1062860610373138.

McNally M, Curtain J, O'Brien KK, et al. Validity of British Thoracic Society guidance (the CRB-65 rule) for predicting the severity of pneumonia in general practice: systematic review and meta-analysis. *Br J Gen Pract.* 2010;60(579):e423–e433. https://doi.org/10.3399/bjgp10X532422.

Medicines & Healthcare Products Regulatory Agency. Medical devices: the regulations and how we enforce them. Available at: https://www.gov.uk/government/publications/report-a-non-compliant-medical-device-enforcement-process/how-mhra-ensures-the-safety-and-quality-of-medical-devices. Accessed 24 May 2020.

Morton S, Igantowicz A, Gnani S, et al. *Describing Team Development Within a Novel GP-Led Urgent Care Centre Model: A Qualitative Study.* British Medical Journal Publishing Group; 2016.

National FGM. Support clinics overview – female genital mutilation (FGM). Available at: https://www.nhs.uk/conditions/female-genital-mutilation-fgm/. Accessed 24 May 2020.

National Institute for Health and Clinical Excellence. Infection: prevention and control of healthcare-associated infections in primary and community care. Available at: https://www.nice.org.uk/guidance/cg139/evidence/control-full-guideline-pdf-185186701. Accessed 24 May 2020.

National Patient Safety Agency. *A risk matrix for risk managers.* Available at: https://www.neas.nhs.uk/media/118673/foi.16.170_-_risk_matrix_for_risk_managers_v91.pdf. Accessed 24 May 2020.

National Quality Board (a). *Human Factors in Healthcare: a Concordat From the National Quality Board*. Available at: https://www.england.nhs.uk/wp-content/uploads/2013/11/nqb-hum-fact-concord.pdf. Accessed May 20, 2020.

National Quality Board (b). Human factors in healthcare. Available at: http://www.england.nhs.uk/ourwork/part-rel/nqb/ag-min/. Accessed 24 May 2020.

NHSE (a). *Clinical Guidelines for Major Incidents and Mass Casualty Events*. Available at: https://www.england.nhs.uk/wp-content/uploads/2018/12/version1-Major_Incident_and_Mass_casualty_guidelines-Nov-2018.pdf. Accessed 20 May 2020.

NHSE (b). About urgent and emergency care. Available at: https://www.england.nhs.uk/urgent-emergency-care/about-uec/. Accessed 24 May 2020.

NHSE (c). Ambulance response programme. Available at: https://www.england.nhs.uk/urgent-emergency-care/improving-ambulance-services/arp/. Accessed 24 May 2020.

NHSE (d). *Building and Strengthening Leadership: Leading With Compassion*. Available at: https://www.england.nhs.uk/wp-content/uploads/2014/12/london-nursing-accessible.pdf. Accessed 24 May 2020.

NHSE (e). Clinically-led review of NHS access standards. Available at: https://www.england.nhs.uk/clinically-led-review-nhs-access-standards/. Accessed 24 May 2020.

NHSE (f). *Integrated Urgent Care Service Specification*. Available at: https://www.england.nhs.uk/wp-content/uploads/2014/06/Integrated-Urgent-Care-Service-Specification.pdf. Accessed 24 May 2020.

NHSE (g). *London Mental Health Response to Major Incidents Pathway for Adult Witnesses*. Available at: https://www.healthylondon.org/wp-content/uploads/2017/10/London-incident-support-pathway-for-adult-witnesses.pdf. Accessed 24 May 2020.

NHSE (h). *MDT Development – Working Toward an Effective Multidisciplinary/Multiagency Team*. Available at: https://www.england.nhs.uk/wp-content/uploads/2015/01/mdt-dev-guid-flat-fin.pdf. Accessed 24 May 2020.

NHSE (i). Mental capacity act. Available at: https://www.nhs.uk/conditions/social-care-and-support-guide/making-decisions-for-someone-else/mental-capacity-act/. Accessed 24 May 2020.

NHSE (j). NHS digital. Available at: https://digital.nhs.uk. Accessed 24 May 2020.

NHSE (k). *NHS England Response to the Specific Duties of the Equality Act: Equality Information Relating to Public Facing Functions*. Available at: https://www.england.nhs.uk/wp-content/uploads/2016/02/nhse-specific-duties-equality-act.pdf. Accessed 24 May 2020.

NHSE (l). NHS long term plan. Available at: https://www.longtermplan.nhs.uk. Accessed 24 May 2020.

NHSE (m). *Serious Incident Framework Supporting Learning to Prevent Recurrence*. Available at: https://www.england.nhs.uk/wp-content/uploads/2015/04/serious-incidnt-framwrk-upd.pdf. Accessed 20 May 2020.

NHSE (n). *Serious Incident Framework Supporting Learning to Prevent Recurrence*. Available at: https://www.england.nhs.uk/wp-content/uploads/2015/04/serious-incidnt-framwrk-upd.pdf. Accessed 24 May 2020.

NHSE (o). *Urgent treatment centres – principles and standards*. Available at: https://www.england.nhs.uk/publication/urgent-treatment-centres-principles-and-standards/. Accessed 24 May 2020.

NHSE and Health Education England. *Integrated Urgent Care/NHS 111 Workforce Blueprint*. Available at: https://www.england.nhs.uk/wp-content/uploads/2018/03/career-of-choice.pdf. Accessed 24 May 2020.

NHS: Education for Scotland. *Clinical Decision Making*. Available at: http://www.effectivepractitioner.nes.scot.nhs.uk/media/254840/clinical%20decision%20making.pdf. Accessed 24 May 2020.

NHS Improvement (a). *Cause and Effect (Fishbone)*. Available at: https://improvement.nhs.uk/documents/2093/cause-effect-fishbone.pdf. Accessed 24 May 2020.

NHS Improvement (b). *Guide to Reducing Long Hospital Stays.* Available at: https://improvement. nhs.uk/documents/2898/Guide_to_reducing_long_hospital_stays_FINAL_v2.pdf. Accessed 24 May 2020.

NHS Improvement (c). *Rapid Improvement Guide to: The 6 As of Managing Emergency Admissions.* Available at: https://improvement.nhs.uk/documents/630/6As-managing-emergency-admissions-RIG.pdf. Accessed 24 May 2020.

NHS Improvement (d). *Root Cause Analysis Using Five Whys.* Available at: https://improvement. nhs.uk/documents/2156/root-cause-analysis-five-whys.pdf. Accessed 20 May 2020.

NHS Improvement (e). *SBAR Communication Tool.* Available at: https://improvement.nhs.uk/ documents/2162/sbar-communication-tool.pdf. Accessed 24 May 2020.

NHS Institute for Innovation and Improvement. The patient experience book: a collection of the NHS institute for innovation and improvement's guidance and support. Available at: https:// www.england.nhs.uk/improvement-hub/wp-content/uploads/sites/44/2017/11/Patient-Experience-Guidance-and-Support.pdf. Accessed 24 May 2020.

NHS Leadership Academy. *Healthcare Leadership Model: The Nine Dimensions of Leadership Behaviour.* Available at: https://www.leadershipacademy.nhs.uk/wp-content/uploads/2014/ 10/NHSLeadership-LeadershipModel-colour.pdf. Accessed 24 May 2020.

Nightingale S, Spiby H, Sheen K, et al. The impact of emotional intelligence in health care professionals on caring behaviour towards patients in clinical and long-term care settings: findings from an integrative review. *Int J Nurs Stud.* 2018a;80:106–117. https://doi.org/10.1016/ j.ijnurstu.2018.01.006.

Nor AM, Davis J, Sen B, et al. The recognition of stroke in the emergency room (ROSIER) scale: development and validation of a stroke recognition instrument. *Lancet Neurol.* 2005;4(11): 727–734. https://doi.org/10.1016/S1474-4422(05)70201-5.

O'Sullivan ED, Schofield SJ. Cognitive bias in clinical medicine. *J R Coll Physicians Edinb.* 2018; 48(3):225–232. https://doi.org/10.4997/JRCPE.2018.306.

Office of the Public Guardian. Safeguarding policy: protecting vulnerable adults. Available at: https://www.gov.uk/government/publications/safeguarding-policy-protecting-vulnerable-adults. Accessed 24 May 2020.

Patient Safety First (a). *Case Example – Elaine Bromiley.* Available at: https://www.patientsafety-first.nhs.uk. Accessed 24 May 2020.

Patient Safety First (b). *The 'How to Guide' for Implementing Human Factors in Healthcare.* Available at: https://www.guysandstthomas.nhs.uk/resources/education-training/sail/reading/ human-factors.pdf. Accessed 24 May 2020.

Peerally MF, Carr S, Waring J, et al. The problem with root cause analysis. *BMJ Qual Saf.* 2017;26(5):417–422. https://doi.org/10.1136/bmjqs-2016-005511.

Primary Care Foundation. Overview: access and urgent care in general practice. Available at: http:// www.primarycarefoundation.co.uk/urgent-care-in-general-practice.html. Accessed 24 May 2020.

Public Health England. Human trafficking: migrant health guide. Available at: https://www.gov. uk/guidance/human-trafficking-migrant-health-guide. Accessed 24 May 2020.

Rapezzi C, Ferrari R, Branzi A. *White Coats and Fingerprints: Diagnostic Reasoning in Medicine and Investigative Methods of Fictional Detectives.* British Medical Journal Publishing Group; 2005.

Reason J. *Human Error: Models and Management.* London: British Medical Journal Publishing Group; 2000.

Royal College of Emergency Medicine (a). Role and establishment of urgent and emergency care networks. Available at: https://www.nhs.uk/NHSEngland/keogh-review/Documents/ Role-Networks-advice-RDs%201.1FV.pdf. Accessed 24 May 2020.

Royal College of Emergency Medicine (b). Time to act – urgent care and A&E: the patient perspective. Available at: https://www.rcem.ac.uk/docs/Policy/CEM8480-Time%20to%20 Act%20Urgent%20Care%20and%20A+E%20the%20patient%20perspective.pdf. Accessed 24 May 2020.

Royal College of Physicians. Improving teams in healthcare. Available at: https://www.rcplondon.ac.uk/projects/improving-teams-healthcare. Accessed 24 May 2020.

Seager L, Smith DW, Patel A, et al. Applying aviation factors to oral and maxillofacial surgery – the human element. *Br J Oral Maxillofac Surg*. 2013;51(1):8–13. https://doi.org/10.1016/j.bjoms.2011.11.024.

Skills for Health. Statutory/mandatory core skills training framework (CSTF). Available at: https://www.skillsforhealth.org.uk/services/item/146-core-skills-training-framework. Accessed 24 May 2020.

Smith M, Higgs J, Ellis E. Factors influencing clinical decision making. In: *Clinical Reasoning in the Health Professions*. 3rd ed./8th ed. (section 2) Sydney: Butterworth-Heinemann; 2008:89–100.

The Faculty of Intensive Care Medicine and Society of Intensive Care. Care guidance on: the transfer of the critically ill adult. Available at: https://www.ficm.ac.uk/sites/ficm/files/documents/2021-10/Transfer_of_Critically_Ill_Adult.pdf. Accessed 24 May 2020.

The Health Foundation. Emergency hospital admissions in England: which may be avoidable and how? Available at: https://www.health.org.uk/publications/emergency-hospital-admissions-in-england-which-may-be-avoidable-and-how. Accessed 24 May 2020.

The King's Fund (a). *Avoiding Hospital Admissions: What Does the Research Evidence Say?* Available at: https://www.kingsfund.org.uk/sites/default/files/Avoiding-Hospital-Admissions-Sarah-Purdy-December2010_0.pdf. Accessed 24 May 2020.

The King's Fund (b). The quality of GP diagnosis and referral. Available at: https://www.kingsfund.org.uk/sites/default/files/Diagnosis%20and%20referral.pdf. Accessed 24 May 2020.

The Primary Care Foundation. The 7 myths of urgent care. Available at: https://www.primary-carefoundation.co.uk/the-7-myths-of-urgent-care.html. Accessed 24 May 2020.

The Royal College of Surgeons of Edinburgh. Exams. Available at: https://www.rcsed.ac.uk/exams. Accessed 24 May 2020.

Thompson M, Vodicka TA, Blair PS, et al. Duration of symptoms of respiratory tract infections in children: systematic review. *BMJ*. 2013:347–f7027. https://doi.org/10.1136/bmj.f7027.

Trimble M, Hamilton P. The thinking doctor: clinical decision making in contemporary medicine. *Clin Med*. 2016;16(4):343–346. https://doi.org/10.7861/clinmedicine.16-4-343.

Tuckey MR, Scott JE. Group critical incident stress debriefing with emergency services personnel: a randomized controlled trial. *Anxiety Stress Coping*. 2014;27(1):38–54. https://doi.org/10.1080/10615806.2013.809421.

Turnbull J, Pope C, Prichard J, et al. A conceptual model of urgent care sense-making and help-seeking: a qualitative interview study of urgent care users in England. *BMC Health Serv Res*. 2019;19(1):481. https://doi.org/10.1186/s12913-019-4332-6.

Vandewaa EA, Turnipseed DL, Cain G. Panacea or Placebo? An evaluation of the value of emotional intelligence in healthcare workers. *J Health Human Serv Adm*. 2016;38(4):438–477.

Various/Oxbridge Solutions Ltd®. *GP Notebook*. https://doi.org/10.1080/10615806.2013.809421. Accessed 1 May 2021.

Wadhera RK, Parker SH, Burkhart HM, et al. Is the "sterile cockpit" concept applicable to cardiovascular surgery critical intervals or critical events? The impact of protocol-driven communication during cardiopulmonary bypass. *J Thorac Cardiovasc Surg*. 2010;139(2):312–319. https://doi.org/10.1016/j.jtcvs.2009.10.048.

Watson A, Gillespie D. *Status and Sanity: The Modern Guide to GP Consulting: Six S for Success*. Abingdon: Radcliffe; 2013.

Windover AK, Boissy A, Rice TW, et al. The REDE model of healthcare communication: optimizing relationship as a therapeutic agent. *J Patient Exp*. 2014;1(1):8–13. https://doi.org/10.1177/237437431400100103.

World Health Organisation (a). Health technologies and medicines. Available at: http://www.euro.who.int/en/health-topics/Health-systems/health-technologies-and-medicines. Accessed 24 May 2020.

World Health Organisation (b). WHO Guidelines for the pharmacological and radiotherapeutic management of cancer pain in adults and adolescents. Available at: https://www.who.int/ncds/management/palliative-care/cancer-pain-guidelines/en/. Accessed 30 January 2021.

World Health Organisation (c). WHO surgical safety checklist. Available at: https://www.who.int/patientsafety/safesurgery/checklist/en/. Accessed 24 May 2020.

ADDITIONAL READING LIST

Association of Ambulance Chief Executives, Joint Royal Colleges Ambulance Liaison Committee. *JRCALC Clinical Guidelines 2019.* 1st ed. Bridgwater: Class Publishing; 2019.

Auerbach PS, Cushing TA, Harris NS. *Auerbach's Wilderness Medicine.* Philadelphia, PA: Elsevier; 2017.

BMJ Military Health, formerly known as Journal of the Royal Army Medical Corps. London: BMJ Publishing. Available at: https://militaryhealth.bmj.com.

Brown SN, Kumar D, James C, et al. *JRCALC Clinical Practice Supplementary Guidelines 2017.* Bridgwater: Class Professional Publishing; 2017.

Care Quality Commission. *Care Quality Commission.* Available at: https://www.cqc.org.uk. Accessed 26 May 2020.

Chambers R, Schmid M, Birch-Jones J. *Digital Healthcare: The Essential Guide.* Oxford, UK: Otmoor Publishing Ltd; 2016.

American Academy of Orthopaedic Surgeons (AAOS). *Critical Care Transport.* Sudbury, MA: Jones and Bartlett Publishers; 2011.

Driscoll PA, Macartney I, Mackway-Jones K, et al. *Safe Transfer and Retrieval: The Practical Approach.* 2nd ed. London: BMJ; 2006.

Ellis D, Hooper M. *Cases in Pre-Hospital and Retrieval Medicine.* London: Elsevier; 2010.

Emergency Medicine Journal. *Emergency Medicine Journal* (Online). London: BMJ Publishing; 2001. Available at: https://emj.bmj.com.

Greaves I, Porter KM. *Oxford Handbook of Pre-Hospital Care.* Oxford: Oxford University Press; 2007.

Healthwatch. *Healthwatch.* Available at: https://www.healthwatch.co.uk. Accessed 26 May 2020.

Hughes R. *Patient Safety and Quality: An Evidence-Based Handbook for Nurses.* Rockville, MD: Agency for Healthcare Research and Quality; 2008.

Johnson C. *Oxford Handbook of Expedition and Wilderness Medicine.* 2nd ed. Oxford: Oxford University Press; 2015.

The Journal of Rural Health. *Journal of Rural Health* (Online). Hoboken, NJ: Wiley;1985. Available at: https://onlinelibrary.wiley.com/journal/17480361.

National Clinical Guideline Centre. Infection: prevention and control of healthcare-associated infections in primary and community care. Available at: https://www.nice.org.uk/guidance/cg139/evidence/control-full-guideline-pdf-185186701. Accessed 26 May 2020.

National Institute for Health and Care Excellence. *Clinical Knowledge Summaries.* Available at: https://cks.nice.org.uk/#?char=A. Accessed 26 May 2020.

NB Medical Education. *Hot Topics GP Update Course.* Bolden Colliery: P&S Medical Education, 2020.

NB Medical Education. *Hot Topics Urgent Care Course.* Bolden Colliery: P&S Medical Education; 2017.

NHSE (a). Clinically-led review of NHS access standards. Available at: https://www.england.nhs.uk/clinically-led-review-nhs-access-standards/. Accessed 26 May 2020.

NHSE (b). NHS England response to the specific duties of the equality act. Available at: https://www.england.nhs.uk/wp-content/uploads/2016/02/nhse-specific-duties-equality-act.pdf. Accessed 26 May 2020.

NHSE (c). Role and establishment of urgent and emergency care networks. Available at: https://www.nhs.uk/NHSEngland/keogh-review/Documents/Role-Networks-advice-RDs%201.1FV.pdf. Accessed 26 May 2020.

NHS Improvement (a). A model for measuring quality care. Available at: https://improvement.nhs.uk/documents/2135/measuring-quality-care-model.pdf. Accessed 26 May 2020.

NHS Improvement (b). NHS improvement. Available at: https://improvement.nhs.uk. Accessed 26 May 2020.

NHS Improvement (c). The patient experience book: a collection of the NHS Institute for Innovation and Improvement's guidance and support. Available at: https://www.england.nhs.uk/improvement-hub/wp-content/uploads/sites/44/2017/11/Patient-Experience-Guidance-and-Support.pdf. Accessed 26 May 2020.

Philpott C, Tassone P, Clark M, Baguley DM. *Bullet Points in ENT: Postgraduate and Exit Exam Preparation.* Stuttgart, Germany: Thieme; 2014.

Phipps O, Lugg J. *Rapid Emergency & Unscheduled Care.* Chichester, UK: Wiley Blackwell; 2016.

Pohwer. NHS complaints advocacy. Available at: https://www.pohwer.net/nhs-complaints-advocacy. Accessed 26 May 2020.

Primary Care Foundation *Urgent Care: A Practical Guide to Transforming Same-Day Care in General Practice.* Available at: https://www.primarycarefoundation.co.uk/images/PrimaryCare Foundation/Downloading_Reports/Reports_and_Articles/Urgent_Care_Centres/Urgent_Care_May_09.pdf. Accessed 26 May 2020.

Puri BK, Treasaden IH. *Emergencies in Psychiatry.* Oxford: Oxford University Press; 2008.

Rabinowitz HK. *Caring for the Country: Family Doctors in Small Rural Towns.* New York, NY: Springer Science and Business Media; 2004.

Rosenorn-Lanng D. *Human Factors in Healthcare. Level One.* Oxford, UK: Oxford University Press; 2015.

Remote and Rural Health (Online). Queensland, Australia: Remote and Rural Health. Available at: http://rrh.org.au.

Scottish Intercollegiate Guidelines Network. *Healthcare improvement Scotland.* Available at: https://www.sign.ac.uk. Accessed: 26 May 2020.

Semple D, Smyth R. *Oxford Handbook of Psychiatry.* Oxford: Oxford University Press, Inc.; 2019.

Simon C, Everitt H, van Dorp F, et al. *Oxford Handbook of General Practice.* 4th ed. Oxford: Oxford University Press; 2014.

The King's Fund. Ideas that change health and care. Available at: https://www.kingsfund.org.uk. Accessed 26 May 2020.

The Patients' Association. *Main Site.* Available at: https://www.patients-association.org.uk. Accessed 26 May 2020.

UK Ambulance Services Clinical Practice Guidelines 2016: Including 2017 Supplementary Guidelines. Class Professional Publishing; 2017. The Joint Ambulance Liaison Committee. JRCALC Clinical Practice Guidelines. Association of Ambulance Chief Executives. Available at https://aace.org.uk/clinical-practice-guidelines/.

Various/Oxbridge Solutions Ltd®. *GP Notebook.* https://gpnotebook.com/en-gb/homepage.cfm. Accessed 1 May 2021.

Wilcock J. *General Practice Today: A Practical Guide to Modern Consultations.* Boca Raton: CRC Press, Taylor & Francis Group; 2018.

Wilderness & environmental medicine. *Wilderness & Environmental Medicine* (Online); 1995. https://www.wemjournal.org

Wyatt JP. *Oxford Handbook of Emergency Medicine.* New York, NY: Oxford University Press; 2012.

Page numbers followed by '*f*' indicate figures and '*t*' indicate tables.